MW01504708

IMMUNITY

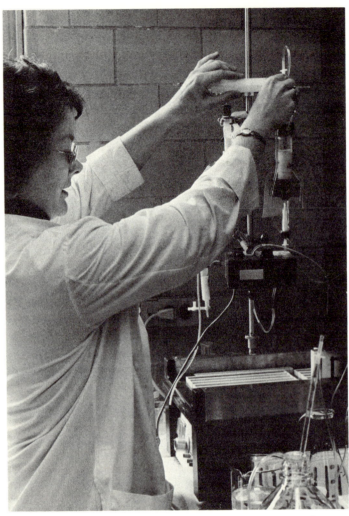

Immunologist Dr. Marian Nau in a laboratory at the National Institutes of Health in Maryland. She is using a technique called affinity chromatography to help reveal how genes control the making of antibodies, kinds of protein that help protect the human body against disease organisms.

IMMUNITY

HOW OUR BODIES
RESIST DISEASE

Joan Arehart-Treichel

HOLIDAY HOUSE • New YORK

PHOTOGRAPHS NOT OTHERWISE CREDITED ARE BY
THE AUTHOR

Library of Congress Cataloging in Publication Data

Arehart-Treichel, Joan.
    Immunity: how our bodies resist disease.

    Bibliography: p. 154
    Includes index.
    SUMMARY: Describes the body's system of antibodies
and how they work to protect against disease. Also
discusses new developments in the field of immunology.
    1. Immunity—Juvenile literature. [1. Immunity]
I. Title. [DNLM: 1. Immunology—Popular works.
QW504 A689i]
QR181.A73   616.07′9   75-30685
ISBN 0-8234-0271-1

For Mother and Daddy,
with thanks
for the brave fighters in my body

ACKNOWLEDGMENTS

I am grateful to the many immunologists who have helped me with this book, especially Dr. Bernard Amos of Duke University; Dr. Philip Leder of the National Institutes of Health; Drs. Charles Hufnagel, Anthony Chung, and Joseph Bellanti of Georgetown University; Dr. Mortimer Bortin of the Mount Sinai Medical Center in Milwaukee; Dr. Raphael Wilson of the Baylor College of Medicine; Dr. Arthur Ammann of the University of California at San Francisco; Dr. Robert J. Sharbaugh of the Medical University of South Carolina.

CONTENTS

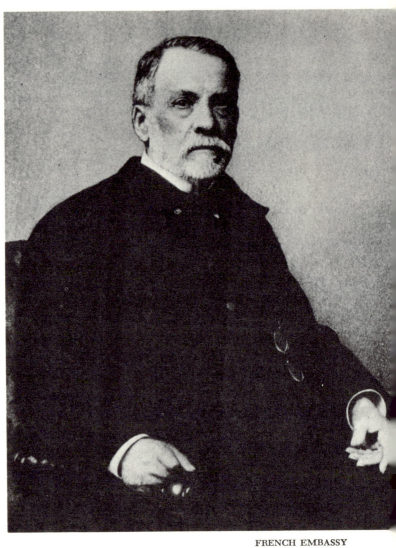

Louis Pasteur, whose great advances in understanding infectious agents and vaccination made modern immunology possible.

1. THE EXPLOSIVE FIELD OF IMMUNOLOGY

Once a year, slim, energetic David Z. of Chatham, New York, and robust David C. of Wallingford, Connecticut, visit each other. Such reunions among young friends are not uncommon. But there is something special about their get-togethers. The two boys became pals in 1968 when they both underwent a similar life-saving operation. Each boy received a bone-marrow transplant that replaced his very weak immune system. . . .

Deborah P. of Chelmsford, Massachusetts, appears to be a typical, fun-loving twelve-year-old. She is bursting with vigor and is good at acrobatics and ballet. But to those who know Debby well, she is a lucky young lady indeed. In 1971 she received a kidney transplant that saved her from a life-threatening kidney disease. . . .

In 1969, a vaccine against German measles was licensed in the United States. Since then, some 55 million American youngsters have received it. Certainly it spares them the discomfort of getting German measles. But more crucial, it is drastically reducing the exposure of pregnant women to German measles. This disease can cause devastating birth defects in unborn children—mental retardation, deafness, heart disease. There were 47,500 infants with birth defects caused by German measles in the United States between 1966 and 1969. In 1974, the number had been reduced to 11,836, thanks to the vaccine.

These are but several examples of how people are benefiting from a field of medical research that is explosive today. The field is immunology—how certain parts of the human body defend it against anything that might be dangerous.

Certainly people's awareness of disease and of the body's efforts to combat it are not new. Back in the fifth century B.C., for example, the Greek physician Hippocrates wrote about the diagnosis and treatment of disease. During the eleventh century, the Chinese and Arabs knew that rubbing smallpox scabs onto a healthy person would help protect him against smallpox. During the eighteenth century, the English physician Edward Jenner built on the knowledge of the Chinese and Arabs and devised a really effective means of smallpox immunization—a smallpox vaccine. During the nineteenth century, the French scientist Louis Pasteur developed his germ theory, thus providing a partial explanation for how the smallpox vaccine works. Thus the stage was set for making vaccines against many other kinds of infectious diseases than just smallpox. And that is precisely what many scientists did during the first half of the twentieth century.

Some progress was also made at that time in identifying some of the parts of our immune system. On the whole, though, a real understanding of how the system works, and how it can be artificially manipulated with vaccines and by other means, did not come until 1950 and onward. There were several reasons. For one, scientists of keen intelligence, such as Sir Frank Macfarlane Burnet of Australia and Sir Peter Medawar of Britain, became interested in immunology around that time. For another, rapid advances were being made in molecular biology—the study of life at its basic chemical level—and these advances encouraged digging into the mysteries of the immune system. Finally, there was generous federal support for this kind of research after World War II.

Men and Women at Microscopes

Today, some 1200 American scientists belong to the American Association of Immunologists. Hundreds can be found in other countries as well. These many investigators are vigorously deciphering the way the immune system works and finding out how it can be manipulated against not only infectious ailments but also against cancer, allergies, and other diseases. These investigators are trying to trick the immune system into letting organ transplants "take"—this is, become attached permanently to the body. They are trying to correct defects

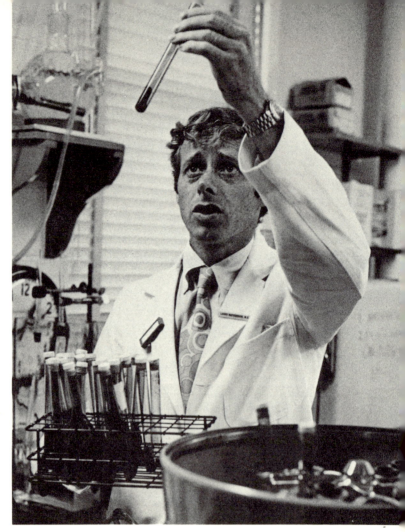

TUFTS-NEW ENGLAND MEDICAL CENTER

Hundreds of scientists throughout the world are trying to find out how immunity works, and how to make it more effective. This is Dr. Larry Nathanson of Tufts-New England Medical Center in Boston. With Dr. David A. Clark he devised a system to monitor immunological changes before, during, and after treatment with BCG, a vaccine made from tuberculosis bacteria that helps defeat certain kinds of cancer.

in the immune system that allow people to become diseased.

In a sense, then, the latter half of the twentieth century is the "golden age of immunology." And in the following chapters we will examine what this age is bringing us, and what went before.

First we'll look at what immunologists now know about how the immune fighters in the human body work. In a sense, they are organized like an army; each carries out its own kind of job, but all the jobs are related. Next we'll examine why the human immune system changes from the moment of conception in the womb through adolescence, adulthood, and up to death. We will see how people vary markedly in the strength of their immune systems, how vaccines got started, and what is now known about the organisms that cause various infectious diseases, including the deadly slow viruses.

We will probe the controversial role of of the immune fighters against cancer, allergies, asthma, and the so-called autoimmune diseases—ailments with exotic names like lupus erythematosus and myasthenia gravis. We will immerse ourselves in the dramatic world of organ transplantation, and of helping youngsters whose immune systems have serious defects (one of them has lived in a germ-free plastic bubble ever since he was born). We shall come to the immune horizon—the great advances that are spilling out of laboratories and clinics month by month—and finally, see what immunologists recommend that each of us do to keep our immune systems strong and healthy.

2. HOW THE IMMUNE FIGHTERS WORK

Have you ever wondered why, on a crisp autumn day, a boy or girl is likely to jump out of bed in the morning? Why he or she rushes off for baseball, horseback riding, or ballet lessons? It's because the brain gives the human body the "go" signal. Then heart, blood vessels, nerves, and muscles get one's body moving.

But there are other parts of the body you may not have thought much about—the parts that rise to defense if one is threatened by bacteria, viruses, or other organisms. They defend one against just about anything that is foreign. They are, of course, the fighters-back in the body—the immune system.

This system extends throughout the body, forming an elaborate, interdependent network of some trillion cells. The cells usually "recognize" the difference between self and nonself. They respond to present events in the view of past ones. But sometimes they make mistakes and turn against friends rather than foes. And sometimes they go so far wrong as to turn upon self, threatening to destroy it.

The source of the immune fighters in the body is bone marrow—spongy connective tissue that fills each bone in the body. Marrow contains cells called stem cells. They are called that because they give rise to different parts of one's blood—red cells, white cells, and platelets. There are white cells that are of the utmost importance in immunity. These white cells are called lymphocytes.

By some mysterious route, lymphocytes travel from bone marrow into a small gland near the heart. This gland is called the thymus. People sometimes mention a food delicacy called sweetbreads. Sweetbreads are thymuses taken from calves. But the thymus has more crucial things to do than be a tasty food. It turn lymphocytes into "T" cells. "T" means that the lymphocytes have passed through the thymus. The gland "trains" inexperienced lymphocytes to become effective fighters. T cells are the major defenders of one's body against disease-causing killers.

A Supermicroscope for an Extra-Small World

Still other lymphocytes leave the bone marrow. But they do not go to the thymus. Instead they go to some other spot where they "learn" to cope with germs and other enemies that attack one. Scientists are not sure where this spot is in people. It may possibly be the liver. But they do know where the spot is in chickens.

It is the bursa of Fabricius, a little gland located at the hind end of the chicken intestine. The cells that come from bone marrow and are processed in the bursa of Fabricius in chickens, and in some other spot in people, are called "B" cells. The "B" stands for either "bursa of Fabricius" or "bone marrow."

A particularly high-powered and sensitive microscope was invented some years ago. It is called the scanning electron microscope. Using this microscope, immunologists at the Memorial Sloan-Kettering Cancer Center and at Rockefeller University looked at B and T cells. They did not look at the cells in a living body, of course, but in slices of tissues that they placed under the microscope. They reported that they saw dramatic differences in the architecture of B and T cells. In their photographs the T cells looked like scoops of ice cream, and B cells looked like balls of fluff with little fingers sticking out all over them.

Then immunologists at the National Cancer Institute attempted to confirm these results. But they were unable to. Their scanning electron microscope pictures show both B and T cells as having short fingers. The NCI scientists admit, though, that the way they pre-

At the top (right), a B cell as seen under a scanning electron microscope, and below it a T cell. It was originally thought that the finger-like projections showing on the B cell were typical for that type of lymphocyte, but later investigation showed that T cells can look the same way under certain conditions. The "fingers," called microvilli, are not necessarily chemical receptors, and their role is still being researched. Each one is not a molecule in itself but is made up of many molecules. MEMORIAL SLOAN-KETTERING CANCER CENTER AND ROCKEFELLER UNIVERSITY

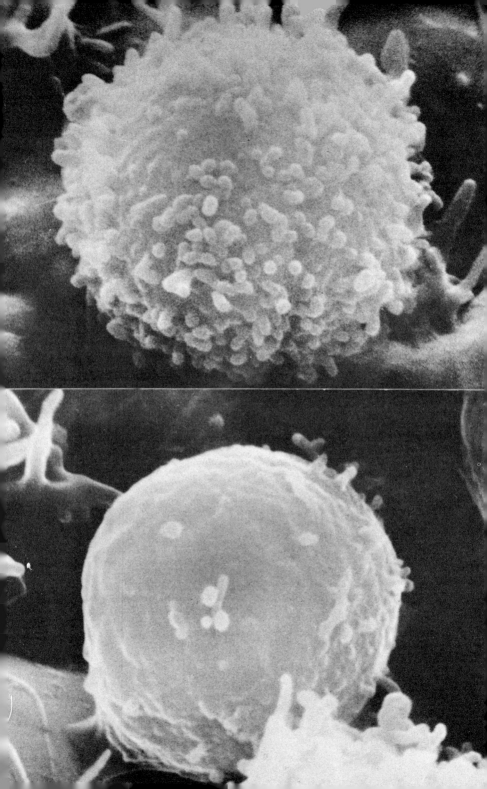

pared the cells for the microscope might account for the differences between their results and those of the other investigators.

Immunologists have also used the scanning electron microscope to count B and T cells and find out their proportions. They estimate that a human body has about four-fifths T cells and one-fifth B cells. However, there are probably billions of each kind of lymphocyte in the body. Counting all of them would be nearly as challenging as counting the stars in the sky.

After T and B cells have been "trained" to fight the enemy, they take up strategic command posts in one's lymph system. This consists of fine tubes full of a colorless fluid called lymph. It is produced by capillaries, the smallest of the blood vessels, and then drains into the lymph system. So in a sense this network is a drainage system. The fine channels come together in lymph nodes—little glands that are found especially in the armpits, behind the ears, and under the jaws. The lymph system also includes larger organs, such as the spleen, which is near the stomach, and masses of lymph tissue, such as the tonsils. The tonsils are estimated to hold some 400 million B and T cells, a rather high figure for two chunks of tissue the size of lima beans.

When T cells meet the enemy, whether it is a bacterium or some other foreign organism, they leave the lymph system and move into the bloodstream. There they surround and destroy the invader. These cells act directly on the enemy. Their action is called "cellular immunity."

But B cells do not attack the enemy directly. They stay in the lymph tissues for the most part and turn out special proteins called antibodies. The antibodies then enter the bloodstream to help the T cells kill the enemy. Immunologists call antibody action "humoral immunity," since "humoral" means "relating to fluids." We will call it antibody immunity, since it seems clearer that way.

The T cells and antibodies don't act alone, though. They also have the help of macrophages. These, like lymphocytes, are a kind of white cell. They are located in many areas of the body.

The T cells, antibodies, and macrophages have still more help from proteins called "complement." These complement proteins come in about a dozen different forms and have various tasks.

Every day of one's life, the immune army is busy fending off an attack. As a young person builds model airplanes, swims, or hunts tadpoles, for instance, it's hard for him or her to realize that a war is actually going on inside him. But if his immunity system has trouble fighting the enemy, he will most decidedly know it. He may break out in a rash or come down with a fever. He may lose his pep and appetite. This means that disease-causing organisms have entered his body and that his immune system is being overwhelmed.

Now let's take a closer, sharper look at all these "specialists" in fighting off organisms that do us damage.

Year by year, even month by month, immunologists

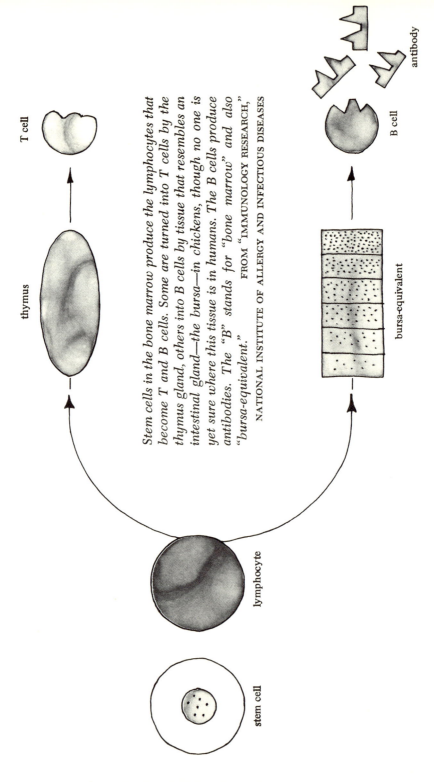

stem cell

lymphocyte

thymus

T cell

bursa-equivalent

B cell

antibody

Stem cells in the bone marrow produce the lymphocytes that become T and B cells. Some are turned into T cells by the thymus gland, others into B cells by tissue that resembles an intestinal gland—the bursa—in chickens, though no one is yet sure where this tissue is in humans. The B cells produce antibodies. The "B" stands for "bone marrow" and also "bursa-equivalent."   FROM "IMMUNOLOGY RESEARCH,"
NATIONAL INSTITUTE OF ALLERGY AND INFECTIOUS DISEASES

are realizing the importance of the thymus. They are learning that the thymus makes chemical mediators— that is, go-betweens—called hormones. It is these hormones that appear to turn stem cells from the marrow into T cells. For instance, when mice were given injections of one of these hormones—thymin—it turned some of their marrow cells into T cells.

Once T cells leave the thymus, they go to other lymph tissues. But they don't necessarily stay in these tissues until enemy organisms "lure" them into the bloodstream. They appear in the blood from time to time as if they were advance scouts keeping a watchful eye out; then they return to the lymph tissues. T cells are long-lived; they can live in the body up to 10 or even 20 years before dividing into new cells. In this way they can keep a long memory, so to speak, of what enemies have entered the body. Then, if these same enemies try to get in again, the T cells will be particularly prepared for another combat with them.

The B cells also move into the bloodstream from time to time. But unlike the T cells, they live only a few days before dividing into new B cells. So their "memory" of old enemies isn't nearly as good as that of the cells altered by the thymus.

T cells usually take on the physically big enemies; antibodies produced by B cells usually go for the smaller ones. But it is becoming more and more evident that T cells and antibodies usually help each other. T cells help antibodies to deal with the smaller organisms; antibodies also participate in killing some of the larger ones.

How do T cells and antibodies get together? There is ample evidence that the T cells are the first to make contact with invading organisms. Then they give off a certain chemical. This substance is thought to contain a piece of the invader. The substance signals the B cells and delivers to them the fragment from the invader's body. The B cells chemically identify the kind of enemy they are up against; then they produce the proper antibodies.

There are little chemical molecules all over the surfaces of T and B cells. These molecules are probably receptors for the invader, or perhaps evidence coming from the invader. Exactly what the receptors are, and how they work, is one of the hottest areas of current immunological research.

The receptors on each B cell, for instance, are probably unique to that cell. With such an arrangement each kind of B cell can "recognize" a specific kind of invader. And only if a B cell recognizes its kind of enemy will it dispatch antibodies to deal with it. But what about T cells? Does each T cell also have receptors that react to only one kind of enemy? Or do they all have the same sort of receptors, and hence react to all invaders? Immunologists aren't sure.

"Fingers" and Molecules

And how about those little finger-like projections? Are they chemical receptors? If they are, why do B cells contact the invader both with their fingers and with the smooth areas of their surfaces? And why is it that T cells are usually smooth on their surfaces, but apparently stick out little fingers when they "see" an invader? Is it because the fingers have receptors for the dangerous organisms? If so, where do T cells hide the fingers if no invader is present? Immunologists are seeking answers to these provocative questions.

What *is* known, however, is that the surfaces of T and B cells change as the temperature changes. So perhaps temperature influences their receptors and their sensitivity to invading organisms. There is also increasing evidence that the chemical receptors on B cells may, in fact, be antibodies. This would not be particularly surprising, because B cells make antibodies. But what is a real shocker is the growing evidence that the chemical receptors on T cells are also antibodies. T cells aren't supposed to make antibodies.

Whether the receptors on B and T cells really are what they seem, a lot is known about the chemistry of antibodies. Scientists have been able to learn a good deal as the substances move along through the blood.

During the early 1960s a British chemist, R. R. Porter, and an American chemist, G. M. Edelman, discovered that antibodies treated with certain chemicals fall to pieces. Drs. Porter and Edelman then started studying the chemistry of these pieces. They found that the fragments are made up of long and short polypeptide chains. These chemical chains are the building bricks of proteins. By 1969 they had figured out the entire chemistry of an antibody. This was the first time for such a feat. And for it the two chemists won the 1972 Nobel Prize for Medicine. This prize is the most distinguished medical research award in the world.

As might be expected, Drs. Porter and Edelman got dozens of other scientists interested in the chemistry of antibodies. And as a result, immunologists now know that there are five different classes of them: IgG, IgM, IgA, IgD, and IgE. The "Ig" stands for "immunoglobulin," a class of proteins of which antibodies are a part.

Although all antibodies are known to be immunoglobulins, we do not yet know whether all immunoglobulins serve as antibodies. In other words, it may turn out that some of the chemical receptors on T and B cells are immunoglobulins, but not necessarily antibodies.

IgG is the most common class of antibody in the bloodstream. IgA is present in blood, but it can also be found in saliva, tears, nasal secretions, and other body fluids. It is good at handling ailments that attack the respiratory tract, such as the common cold. IgM antibodies are located in the blood; they are known to be effective killers. Although IgD has been found in blood, its specific biological role is yet to be made clear. There are very low levels of IgE antibodies in blood; that is, unless one suffers from allergies. IgEs are known to make allergies worse, not better. This behavior is contrary to antibodies' usual good-guy role.

IgGs, IgDs, and IgEs consist of two short polypeptide chains (light chains) and two long ones (heavy chains). IgMs are made up of five of these units. This means that each of their units contains two light chains and

Antibodies vary in form, as explained in the text. This picture shows the chainlike molecules, or "chains," of which they are made. The IgG, IgD, and IgE chains, for instance, consist of two short ("light") and two long ("heavy") chains; the IgM consists of five such units. "Serum IgA" refers to that found in the blood's serum; "secretory IgA" refers to that found in body secretions such as saliva and tears.

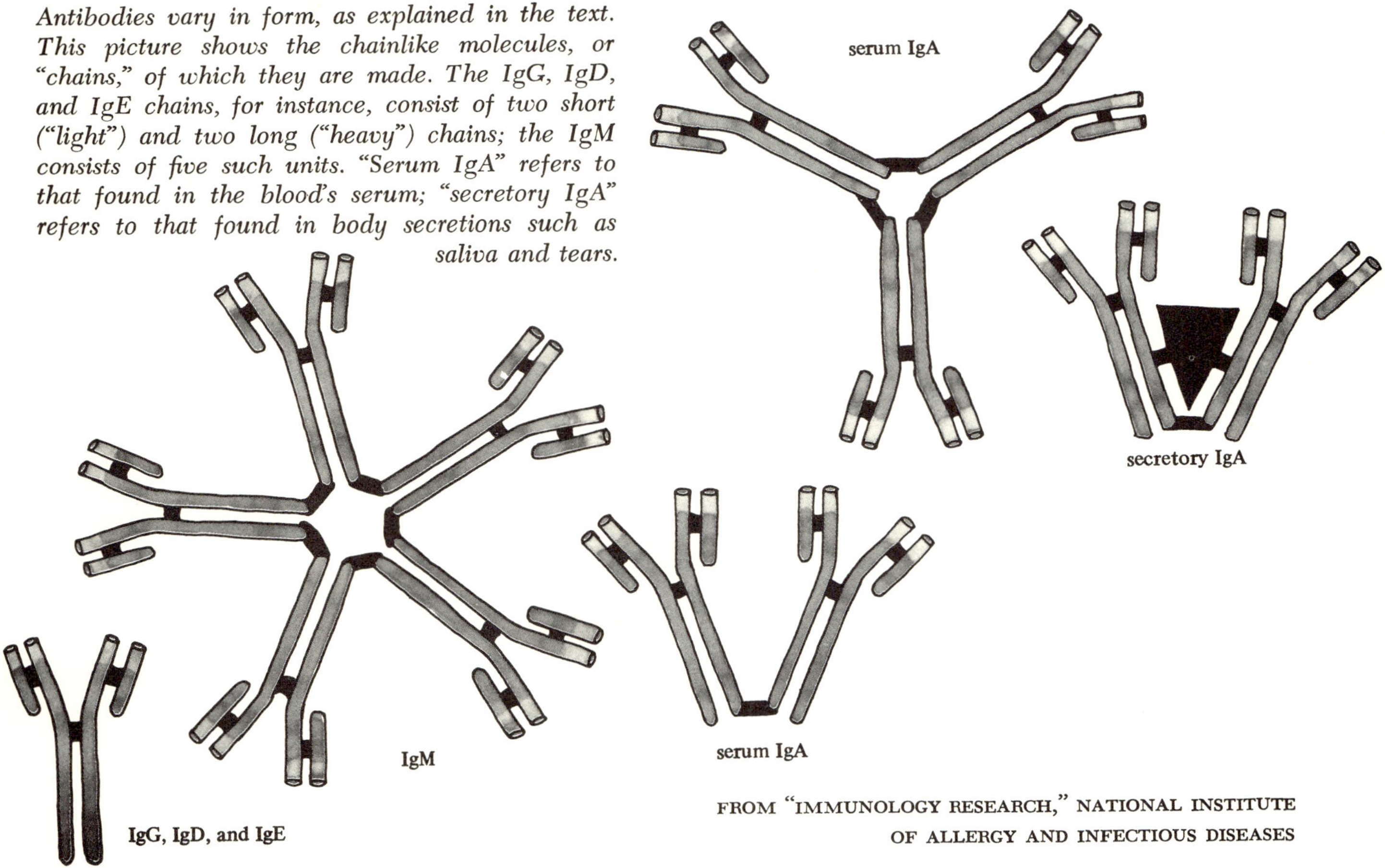

secretory IgA

serum IgA

serum IgA

IgM

IgG, IgD, and IgE

FROM "IMMUNOLOGY RESEARCH," NATIONAL INSTITUTE OF ALLERGY AND INFECTIOUS DISEASES two heavy chains. So altogether they have ten short and ten long chains held in a ring. IgA in the blood consists of one, two, or three units. IgA in body fluids is made up of two units joined by a special link known as the "secretory piece."

When an antibody attacks an invader—which is called an antigen by immunologists—its light and heavy chains make contact with it. The ends of the chains are known as the variable regions. It is these regions that are adapted to just one particular kind of antigen. The other parts of the chains are known as the constant regions. This means they are the same from one antibody to another.

It's very impressive to realize that one's body has a different kind of B cell to fight each antigen it might ever come into contact with; the number of chemical adaptations that occurred during the evolution of human beings over millions of years must have been enormous. As we have seen, each type of B cell makes the kind of antibody that is needed to fight a specific antigen. Thus, when a B cell is alerted by a T cell chemical that its kind of enemy is attacking, the B cell promptly makes hundreds of thousands of one kind of antibody. These substances are able to cope exclusively with this enemy. Some immunologists view a variable region of an antibody as a sort of lock for a specific key, or antigen. Each antibody can interlock with one kind of invader, and with that kind only.

How does a B cell make a particular kind of antibody? Immunologists now know that they are made on little structures called ribosomes. (These are the same structures that are used to make other kinds of proteins as well.) But the reason antibody production is started at all is that some of the genes in the cell ordered it.

Genes and Antibodies

Genes are the genetic material of life. They are present in the nucleus of each cell. Each human cell is estimated to have 100,000 genes. And that includes each B cell. How many of these genes are involved in ordering the production of an antibody? This is a question that has baffled immunogeneticists for some years now. However, they are making some progress in answering it.

They have learned, for instance, that each B cell probably uses three genes to make the constant region of each polypeptide chain that goes into an antibody. Each antibody has two kinds of constant regions: those on heavy chains and those on light chains, so the B cell probably uses a total of six genes. How many genes are involved in making the variable regions of the chains? The answer is not yet known. The variable regions of an antibody are identical, so it's possible that only one gene is required.

And then there is the question of how many genes are needed to put the constant region and variable region of each chain together. And how many are needed to package all the polypeptide chains into one antibody? Even the most sophisticated instruments now available to immunologists are hard pressed to provide the answers.

All these questions are especially challenging because,

while genes can be seen under a very powerful microscope, they all look much the same, like tiny beads. So
immunogeneticists must learn about them and their
functions mostly by nonvisual techniques.

Research into the genes that code for—direct the
manufacture of—antibodies is challenging also because
it has destroyed a former belief—that only one gene
codes for a whole polypeptide chain. Investigation has
shown that each polypeptide chain that goes into an
antibody requires at least two genes, and probably
more. Philip Leder of the National Institutes of Health
is one of the scientists who has helped destroy the classical concept. "Antibodies," he declares, "are strange and
unique protein molecules."

Immunogenetics also causes immunologists to ponder
this tough question: Do all B cells contain the same
genes for constant antibody regions, but contain different genes for variable antibody regions? It's quite possible that all B cells have the same genes for constant
regions because these regions are the same from one
antibody to another. But it's harder to say whether all
B cells have the same genes for variable regions, because
the variable regions change from one antibody to another. In other words, if one gene were needed to code
for each variable region, each B cell would need at least
a million genes to code for all possible variable regions
—that is, for all possible enemies. Yet the B cell would
need only one of these genes to make the kind of variable regions it makes.

So it's unlikely that each B cell contains genes for all

variable regions. It's more likely that each contains only the gene or genes it needs to make its particular kind of variable region.

Immunologists aren't studying just those genes that make antibodies. They are also looking at genes that are involved in other immune products and functions. They now know that each T cell, as well as each B cell, may contain dozens of such genes. And they know that these so-called immune-response genes are located on several different chromosomes. Chromosomes are the structures in the center of the cell that contain genes. There are 46 chromosomes in each of the B and T cells. (In fact, there are normally 46 chromosomes in every human cell except for sperm cells and egg cells, which have 23 each.) The chromosome in B and T cells that is especially rich in immune-response genes is the Number Six chromosome.

Immunogeneticists are just starting to get an idea of what immune-response genes do. They know, for instance, that the genes that control the recognition of antibodies are not those that control their production. They think—although they are not positive—that some of the immune-response genes make the chemical receptors on the surfaces of B and T cells.

On the whole, they have vastly more to learn about the functions and actual products of various immune-response genes. And surely as they learn more, the exact functions of receptors on the surfaces of B and T cells should become clearer. And so should the chemical interactions between antibodies and antigens. It's ironic that we are dead-sure of enemy interactions with B cells, T cells and antibodies but still far from sure just how these interactions take place.

Many immunologists are busy trying to better understand interactions between T cells, B cells, antibodies, and enemy invaders. But other immunologists are focusing on the macrophages and complement proteins that help T cells, B cells, and antibodies.

Macrophages play a major role in immune defense and in the disposal of invaders. Immunologists have known this for a long time. Still, they have many questions about where macrophages come from. And they still want to know a lot about the *how* of their fighting abilities.

Macrophages, it seems, have their origin in bone marrow, as T and B cells do. And macrophages too are a kind of white cell. But unlike T cells, macrophages are not "trained" for combat in the thymus, and unlike B cells, are not trained for combat in some unknown hideaway. Primitive forms of macrophages called monocytes simply seem to leave bone marrow. Then the monocytes roam around in the bloodstream and somewhere along the way mature into macrophages.

Many of the macrophages in one's body are swimming in the blood. But many others, for unknown reasons, leave it and settle in other tissues. These include the liver, lungs, kidneys, bone joints, mouth, and lymph tissues.

There seem to be two ways that macrophages help fight off invaders. One is through serving as a first line

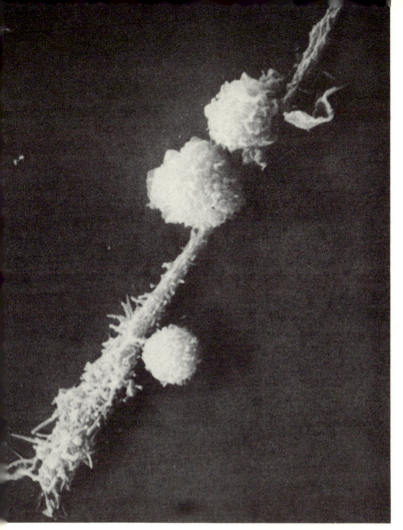

This is a macrophage (stick-shaped) and three small lymphocytes—all forms of white blood cells—as seen by the electron microscope. Macrophages are ordinarily round but this one became stretched out in the course of its activities against invading organisms. Macrophages "collar" some of the organisms and take them to B cells, then engulf and digest the rest of them.

of defense; the second is by acting on the command of T cells.

When macrophages serve as a first line of defense, it's often "up front" in one's body—in lungs, skin, or bloodstream. They first capture some of the invaders alive, then conduct them to B cells, which produce the proper antibodies against them. The macrophages then start gobbing up the rest—engulfing them in their own protoplasm. Once the invaders are inside the macrophages, large protein molecules go to work on them. The proteins, called lysosomes, act like mammoth garbage disposals. They chemically chomp and grind until the invaders are in bits.

The macrophages are not always the first to sound an alarm, though. Many times it is T cells. And when T cells are first, they then alert B cells and macrophages. The T cells order the macrophages to move to the site of the invasion. The cells apparently let the macrophages know where the site is by hanging a chemical signal on the invaders. Macrophages also recognize the site of invasion because they "sense" antibodies fighting the invaders. The macrophages then move into the battle. They attack the invaders with cannonballs of lysosomal enzymes. Macrophages are killer cells; enzymes are their weapons.

Complement: the Protein Backup

The battlefield is already cluttered enough with invaders, T cells, antibodies, and macrophages; but still other troops of the immune army get into the action. They are the complement brigade.

This group consists of from 9 to 11 proteins. These are made in the spleen, lymph nodes, liver, intestines, and lungs. They may even be made by macrophages. The various complement proteins then go into the bloodstream. There is evidence that a certain complement protein Number Three helps T cells alert B cells to an attack. There is also evidence that B cells have chemical receptors on their surfaces that receive messages from complement proteins.

No matter how B cells are alerted about an invasion, they make antibodies, which lock chemically into the invaders. They pull the invaders together into clumps. This way it's hard for the invaders to spread throughout the body and multiply. The complement proteins are also known to communicate with the antibodies and macrophages about the invaders.

In military terms, the complement brigade is a search-and-destroy operation. It proceeds from reconnaissance to deployment to attack. The following is an example of a typical attack involving complements.

Complement Number One attaches itself to an antibody. Number One then joins complement Number Four, and the two release a substance called C-kinin. This substance leads to a swelling of the tissues containing the attack. Complements Number Four and Number Two then uncover Number Three. This latter chemically attacks the invader. At the same time it also makes contact with a mast cell. These special cells, located throughout the body but especially under the skin, release substances called anaphylatoxin and histamine. They lead to inflammation of the tissues being attacked.

Complement Number Three also calls on macrophages to swallow the invaders. In addition it rallies complements Five, Six, and Seven. These call for more macrophages. Numbers Eight and Nine attack invaders and help macrophages destroy them.

An entire immune system, then, uses many cells and proteins as checks and balances. It uses everything it has for signals, countersignals, and duplicate defenses. In a sense it works like those safeguards the government has developed to keep any army mistake from triggering a nuclear attack. It takes more than one signal from more than one immunity group to fire a missile. The complexity and sophistication of the immune system is almost overwhelming.

There is one sobering point to remember, though. Immune fighters do their very best to protect a person every day of his or her life. But their ability to do so isn't the same at all stages of one's life. And the system may be stronger in one person than in another. Let's look at how an immune army is ever changing and why it may not be the same from one human being to another.

3. IMMUNITY: UP AND DOWN— AND STRICTLY PERSONAL

The first nine months of life are like a fast-paced movie thriller. A sperm and an egg join in conception. The fertilized egg divides into two cells, four cells, eight cells, and so on. By the fifth day of life it consists of 50 cells. By the seventh day it attaches itself to the mother's womb. By the fourth week it is about the size of one's fingernail and starting to look like a baby. By the end of the second month it is a boy or girl. By the fourth and fifth months it's turning, twisting, somersaulting, and kicking its mother in the abdomen. In the ninth month (ordinarily) it pops into the world, a wriggling, red-faced little infant.

We all made this transition in the womb. Life in the womb is such a marvelous experience, it's a shame that none of us can remember what it was like!

Scientists are using fancy techniques to spy on this early life. They are learning more fascinating things about it all the time. One of these things is that the immune system starts developing early. It seems to begin as early as eight weeks after conception.

As the unborn baby's bones form, so does its bone marrow. As its marrow forms, it gives rise to stem cells. These cells make lymphocytes. By the eighth week, some of the lymphocytes travel to the baby's developing thymus. There they become T cells. By the twelfth week the T cells start to give immune protection.

Other lymphocytes leave the infant's bone marrow. They travel to the unknown "training" area and become B cells. This training area may be the baby's developing liver. B cells have been found in the liver some 12 weeks after conception. Also at 12 weeks, B cells have been found in the spleen and blood. And the B cells start making antibodies; IgM, IgG, and IgE antibodies have been noted at that time. However, the synthesis of IgA antibodies does not seem to start until seven and a half months after conception. And the making of IgD antibodies doesn't seem to start until after birth.

Not much is known about the development of macrophages before birth. But complement proteins seem to be made as early as 12 weeks.

Immunity in the Womb and Out

For the most part, then, the immunity setup is developing by the twelfth week after conception. But this does not mean that it is completely arranged or can offer full protection. For this reason some of the mother's antibodies cross the membrane screen separating her and her baby. This screen is called the placenta. The maternal antibodies that protect the unborn baby seem to be mostly IgG and some IgE.

A human embryo five weeks old, shown inside its transparent protective sac, the amnion. The feathery-looking tissue attached to the womb is the placenta, through which nourishment comes to the embryo from the mother, and wastes are removed. Blocking antibodies in the placenta apparently serve to protect the embryo from the mother's ordinary antibodies; otherwise the embryo would tend to be rejected as if it were a transplanted organ.

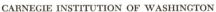

CARNEGIE INSTITUTION OF WASHINGTON

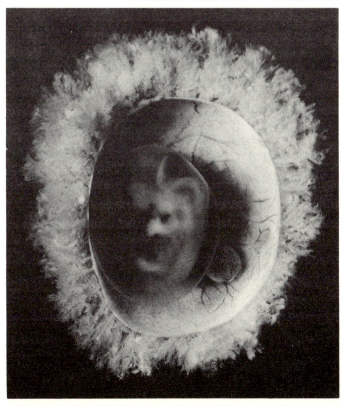

The unborn baby's development in the womb raises a fascinating question about immunity. A baby is half its father and half its mother, genetically speaking. So why don't the mother's immune fighters view the baby in her womb as something foreign? Why don't they consider it an enemy and try to reject it?

Scientists in Dallas, Texas, are trying to answer this question. They grafted unborn animals to unconventional sites of their mothers' bodies. Even so, the unborn animals were not rejected immunologically. So the scientists concluded that the placenta, which is part of the unborn animal, has a special kind of antibody on it, called a blocking antibody. These special chemicals protect the unborn animal from the mother's antibodies and the rest of her immune fighters. So unborn babies may have blocking antibodies to protect them from maternal rejection.

However, once in a while a mother's immune system does get confused. It attacks the unborn baby. In other words, immune tolerance breaks down. And when this happens, the life of the mother and baby may be endangered. The condition is called toxemia of pregnancy.

Fortunately toxemia—a poisoned condition—is not common. Most of the time mothers and their unborn babies coexist peacefully in close physical contact.

By the time a baby is born, its immune system is fairly well developed. But it is still not mature. The antibodies and T cells are sometimes able to kill viruses, bacteria, and other enemies—but not always. Its complement proteins are not yet full-fledged fighters, nor are its macrophages yet able to destroy invaders.

Luckily the baby receives added immune protection from its mother. This protection comes from antibodies she gave it before birth. This extra protection also comes from her milk if she breast-feeds her baby. Mother's milk is rich in IgA antibodies. It may contain other immune fighters as well.

When a baby is born, it has a fairly large thymus. The thymus is about the size of an ordinary clay marble. The thymus helps the baby build up a battalion of T cells. But the thymus also appears to fulfill another function. It seems to help the infant mature sexually.

Two Swiss researchers removed the thymuses from newborn female mice. A few days later these mice and other mice that still had thymuses were examined for sexual development. The mice without thymuses were retarded in sexual growth. The mice with thymuses developed normally. It is probably the hormones in the thymus that assist in sexual development.

Meanwhile the infant's immune fighters are getting tougher and tougher. At three months after birth, they are stronger than at birth. At seven months, they are tougher than at three; and so on. By the time a baby is two years old, its immunity system is about as tough as that of older children, adolescents, and adults.

Growing Older

However, it is during adolescence that the immune army reaches its peak. If a girl or boy is anywhere between 10 and 17, the antibodies can fight enemies off better than at any other time of life. So can the B cells,

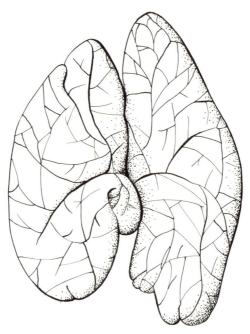

A wonderful organ is the thymus. It is located at the base of the heart, behind the sternum, the bony chest part that connects the upper seven pairs of ribs. It chemically "teaches" T cells, the body's principal defenders, to ward off disease. Its other possible functions are somewhat uncertain. This is how the thymus of a two-year-old child looks.

the T cells, the macrophages, and the complement proteins. The thymus is about as large as it ever has been, and about as large as it will ever be. During adolescence a thymus shrinks.

It may seem strange that one's immunity is at its peak now. Other parts of the body have not reached their peak yet—say, sexual organs and muscles and general physical strength. But it's true. Parts of a human being are old while other parts are young. A body is ever changing.

Of course, the immune fighters are still pretty tough when one reaches his twenties and thirties. But as he moves into the forties, fifties, and sixties, they get tired. They can't fight then with the same energy they used to.

Most persons over age 60 have two small lobes of fat for a thymus. Their spleen and lymph nodes have shrunk. Their T cells, antibodies, B cells, macrophages, and complement proteins have all begun to falter.

It's hardly a surprise, then, that older people, like newborns, are more open to diseases than are individuals of in-between ages. The newborn's immune army has not reached its peak. The older person's immune army is past its prime. As an apparent result, cancer, heart disease, and other ailments usually strike in one's later years.

As you might expect, the decline of the immune system with age intrigues scientists. They are trying to understand why it happens. Is it because the thymus shrinks? Or is it because this gland stops making T cells? Or is there a decrease in stem cells in bone marrow? One scientist believes the weakening is the result of a decline in thymus hormones with age. He treated spleen cells with thymus hormones; they made the spleen cells look and act more youthful.

Some immunologists believe that general aging is the result of a breakdown in the immune system. Aging may be the result of T cells' wearing out. This is the theory of Macfarlane Burnet, one of the granddaddies of twentieth-century immunology. However, two investigators at the Medical College of Georgia have another opinion. Their opinion is that abnormal immunological activity blocks the normal duplication of cells.

They have found that cells from an unborn baby will double 50 times in tissue culture. But cells from older persons double far fewer times. The reason that the cells from older persons do not double very well is that they are blocked. Certain drugs that unblock this cell duplication are the same drugs that suppress the immune system. So they suspect that some breakdown in the body's immune system somehow blocks cell replication. And this blockage leads to aging.

So the immune system changes with chronological aging. But it also changes with the hours, days, weeks, and seasons. It does this no matter what one's age is.

In rats, various physical yardsticks—though not all—are precisely 12 hours out of phase with ours, since they are nocturnal animals. Rats' antibodies peak around 3-4 A.M. and drop to a low about 9-10 P.M. Two Arkansas researchers, Drs. John Pauly and Lawrence Scheving, think therefore (but with proper scientific caution) that human antibodies probably peak about 9-10 P.M. and drop to a low around 3-4 A.M. (Since these hours are only estimates, the investigators prefer to say merely "early evening hours" and "early morning hours.") So one might conclude that people's ability to fight off disease is in top form in the evening and weaker early in the morning; and that if we exert ourselves when our immune fighters are more vulnerable, we are more likely to get sick.

There is, in fact, evidence that this is the case. Students staying up to the crack of dawn studying for exams, persons working during the early morning hours, and international travelers who miss sleep because of changes in time zones are known to be more susceptible to colds and other infections than those who sleep during the early morning hours.

No one else in the world has an immune system exactly like anyone else's. Not even one's mother, father, sisters, or brothers duplicate one's own. There are several reasons for this uniqueness. One reason is a genetic one: each person is a *blend* of the immune-response genes handed down by his parents. These genes determine how strong or weak the new immune system will be. Both animal and human studies prove this.

Antibodies are known to vary in chemical composition from person to person, and these variations are under genetic control. Such variations in antibodies are known as allotypes. They have been identified and classified into several groups. One group is confined to the heavy chains of IgE antibodies. The other group of variations can be found in the light chains of all antibody classes.

Tonsils, as we mentioned before, contain many B and T cells. They play a big role in cellular immunity against measles, flu, polio, the common cold, and other infectious diseases. Immunologists at Georgetown Medical

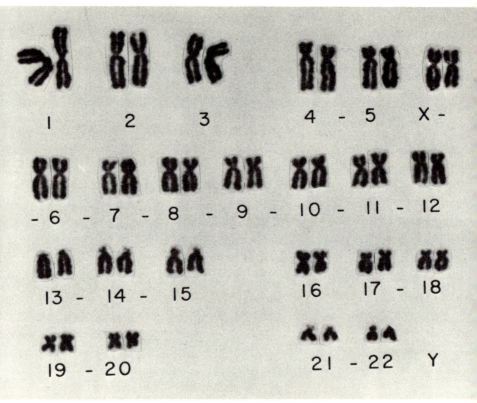

1   2   3   4 - 5   X -

- 6   - 7   - 8   - 9   - 10 -   11 -   12

13 -   14 -   15   16   17 -   18

19 -   20   21 - 22   Y

THE NATIONAL FOUNDATION—MARCH OF DIMES

No one's immune system is exactly like anyone else's, partly because the parents' genes are blended in him or her. Genes are contained in chromosomes, shown in this karyotype, or photographic diagram, much enlarged by a microscope. There are two X chromosomes here and no Y chromosome, indicating that they came from a female; one X and one Y would indicate a male. Chromosomes are found in the nucleus of every human body cell (except red blood cells when these cells mature); their study has advanced not only immunology but many other areas of biology and medicine as well.

School in Washington, D.C., studied persons aged five to 22 years who were having their tonsils removed for one reason or another. The immunologists took lymphocytes from their blood just before the operations. Then after the tonsils were removed, lymphocytes were taken from these. The immunologists found that the lymphocytes from the blood and tonsils of each person were equally good fighters. But the lymphocytes from one person were not as strong as those from another. This result suggests that some of the persons had been genetically endowed with strong immune systems and others had not.

Other investigators studied 100 children for the ability of their antibodies to fight off bacteria. They found that some of the children had 10 times better antibody fighters than did others. These results also suggest genetic differences.

These same scientists studied rabbits antibody responses to bacteria. They found that some of the animals made more antibodies than others did. They then bred the rabbits with lots of antibodies to each other. They also bred the rabbits with fewer antibodies to each other. Almost all of the offspring of the first group had large quantities of antibodies. Almost all of the offspring of the second group had fewer antibodies. The scientists conclude: "It would appear that the total amount of antibody that can be produced is under genetic control."

A Minnesota immunogeneticist believes that one reason some people age faster than others is that they have inherited different immune defenses. He studied strains of naturally long-lived mice and strains of naturally short-lived mice. Only the latter group showed a decline in antibody production before they lived out their normal life span. "My work," the scientist reports, "shows that mice, and probably people as well, are not born with the same immune defenses. There are mice and people who are old when they are young. And there are mice and people who are young when they are old."

Inherited individual differences in immune strength make for vast differences in the ease of developing diseases. Some persons have been found to lack, or to be deficient in T cells, B cells, particular antibodies, or other immunity components. And sure enough, when they do not have these immune fighters, or enough of them, they get diseases that other people can usually fight off.

The Case of Peter

A prime, and very sad, example of this fact is the case of a 16-year-old boy from Ohio—we'll call him Peter J. Smith. He came down with what appeared to be infectious mononucleosis. "Mono" is a rather common viral disease among adolescents who get run down from too many activities. Peter coughed. He had a scratchy sore throat. He was dead tired. He went to bed. Most mono victims recover by resting in bed. Peter didn't. He got worse. His parents called the hospital, and an ambulance took him to the hospital. Once at the hospital, Peter was tested for his immune defenses.

The hospital staff found that his lymphocytes and macrophages were low in number. Blood tests showed the presence of herpes virus, which is known to cause mono. They gave Peter different kinds of treatment to bolster his immune fighters against the virus. Peter's immune army rallied. But then it declined again. He died on his eighth day in the hospital.

This tragic and true story brings home all too vividly the importance of immunity in fending off death-causing diseases. But it also shows up something about his immune defenses. The doctors and nurses who cared for Peter found later that though Peter had high levels of IgG, IgM, and IgA antibodies, he could not make antibodies that were specifically tailored to the mono virus.

In other words, it looked as if Peter lacked that one-in-a-million kind of antibody that is needed to fight off the mono virus. What's more, his T cells weren't up to par. And the doctors and nurses discovered that three of Peter's cousins had also died from mono. So they were now convinced that Peter had died because of genetic immune deficiencies.

So the strength of one's immune army depends, to a large degree, on what one has inherited from one's parents. It can also depend on one's sex: females tend to be more resistant to diseases than males. This resistance may be the result of having tougher immune armies or it may be the result of having protective sex hormones.

The vigor of one's immune system may be influenced by still a third factor: race. In other words, one's immune strength depends also on the kind of immune strength his ancestors have built up during the past hundreds of years. Some races can fight back strongly at a certain disease and some cannot.

Back during the sixteenth century, for instance, the Spanish conqueror Cortes used only a few hundred men to conquer thousands of warlike and brave Mexican Aztecs. How did Cortes do this? He made allies with the Indians and also betrayed them behind their backs. But what really helped him bring off a victory was that the Aztecs were struck by an epidemic of smallpox. The Spaniards had brought the smallpox with them from Spain. Their immune systems "knew" smallpox and to some extent could cope with it. But the Indians' immune systems had never encountered smallpox before and were not adapted to coping with it. The Indians' susceptibility to smallpox was so great that the disease toppled them more effectively than swords.

Environmental factors can also have a bearing on the strength of one's immune system. The food a mother eats while carrying a developing child in her womb, for instance, probably has an impact on its immune system. Immunologist Paul Newberne, together with his team at the Massachusetts Institute of Technology, has found that if mother rats are given only marginal levels of protein to eat, their offspring are born with weakened immune systems and resistance to infections. They also found that if mother rats were given marginal levels of the B vitamins, the same thing happened.

And the food eaten as an infant, and as a child or a

teenager, probably also influences the immune system. When protein was added to the diets of a group of children, their susceptibility to infections dropped by a third. Burned children are particularly open to infections. When they were fed a lot of protein, their infections went away.

Still other environmental factors can influence the strength of the immune system. For instance, the viruses, bacteria, and other pathogens one has come into contact with. If the immune army has overcome certain enemies in the past, it will remain primed for action against them and will almost certainly win out. This protective device is known as "immune memory."

4. IMMUNITY AND THE SCOURGE OF INFECTIOUS DISEASES

Ever since the glorious age of Greece, people have been aware that the body protects itself against infectious diseases. During the plague of Athens, only those few persons who recovered from the disease were able to nurse the sick and bury the dead. During the fifteenth century the word "immunity" arose to describe the exemption from military service of men who had survived the Black Plague. These men could be drafted as nurses for plague victims because they would not get the plague again. The reason for this resistance, as we know today, is that once a person's immune system overcomes a particular disease, he will probably not fall prey to the disease again.

Even as early as the eleventh century, however, people were starting to realize something else about immunity and infectious diseases. This was that if a person was exposed to the sores of someone with a particular disease, he would probably not get the disease. In fact the Chinese and Arabs made an effort to inhale the scabs of victims of smallpox. They hoped that such exposure would protect them against smallpox.

During the eighteenth century, Lady Mary Wortley Montagu was the wife of the English ambassador to the Ottoman Empire (now Turkey). Lady Montagu learned about the Arabs' immunizing themselves against smallpox by inserting bits of smallpox scabs into the bloodstream. She had her own son immunized the same way. When she returned to England she tried to convert the English to the practice.

Certainly there was a need for it. Thirty out of every 100 persons were coming down with smallpox, and those who didn't die from the disease were left with horrible scars on their faces. The clergy thundered at Lady Montagu for interfering with the designs of God. Some people accused her of experimenting on her own child. But Lady Montagu was a strong person. She was also an aristocrat, and powerful. She arranged that six criminals be exposed to smallpox scabs. The exposure protected them from smallpox. She arranged that orphan children be immunized in the same way. It worked as well. Then England's Princess Caroline had her two daughters exposed to smallpox scabs. Smallpox immunization was widely received. It spread rapidly throughout England and western Europe.

This massive immunization against smallpox prevented thousands of deaths. It most likely was one reason for the vast increase in population during the

AN

INQUIRY

INTO

THE CAUSES AND EFFECTS

OF

THE VARIOLÆ VACCINÆ,

A DISEASE

DISCOVERED IN SOME OF THE WESTERN COUNTIES OF ENGLAND,

PARTICULARLY

GLOUCESTERSHIRE,

AND KNOWN BY THE NAME OF

THE COW POX.

BY EDWARD JENNER, M. D. F. R. S. &c.

——— — QUID NOBIS CERTIUS IPSIS
SENSIBUS ESSE POTEST, QUO VERA AC FALSA NOTEMUS.

LUCRETIUS.

London:

PRINTED, FOR THE AUTHOR,

BY SAMPSON LOW, N°. 7, BERWICK STREET, SOHO:

AND SOLD BY LAW, AVE-MARIA LANE; AND MURRAY AND HIGHLEY, FLEET STREET

1798.

The title page of one of the world's most valuable books, Edward Jenner's announcement of his method of preventing smallpox by vaccination. Putting the principles from this book into practice for over 150 years, physicians have been able to save millions of human lives that would formerly have been claimed by this disease.

eighteenth century. And this increase helped set the stage for the Industrial Revolution and the urban civilization in which we now live.

"*I Cannot Get Smallpox*"

Smallpox immunization was further refined toward the end of the eighteenth century. One bright spring day in 1796, an English country physician named Edward Jenner chatted with a dairymaid. He learned that she, like many dairymaids and farmers, had been accidentally infected with cowpox, which is a mild disease. "For this reason," she told Jenner, "I cannot get smallpox."

The dairymaid's remark gave Jenner an idea. He took pus from a cowpox sore and inserted it under the skin of a healthy eight-year-old boy. Later Jenner exposed the boy to smallpox. And as he hoped, the child was immune to this dread disease. Cowpox immunization as a means of protecting against smallpox was well received by physicians, after some resistance. By the end of the eighteenth century some 100,000 persons had undergone the procedure.

However, there was something that the Chinese, the Arabs, Lady Montagu, and Jenner didn't know. It was why immunization with smallpox scabs or with cowpox sores protected people against smallpox. The first step toward explaining this mysterious phenomenon came in 1877. A French chemist named Louis Pasteur discovered that germs can cause disease. He found out that various infectious diseases are caused by organisms such as bacteria. Pasteur coined a name for the technique of using such organisms to confer immune protection. He called it a vaccination, from the Latin word for "cow," which is *vacca*. This name was in honor of Jenner's contributions.

Pasteur also learned how to take fierce organisms and change them into weak organisms. In this way the organisms could be used to induce protection. But they would not be so likely to cause active disease.

A second step toward explaining the phenomenon of immunization came in 1894. A German chemist named Richard Pfeiffer discovered that there are proteins in the blood that fight invading germs. These proteins were later named antibodies. And the germ invaders came to be called antigens. Pitting one "anti" against another is not at all logical. It has disturbed immunologists for years. But still the name has stuck.

So the stage was set for explaining how vaccination works. An infectious germ, or a weakened version of it, is injected into a person. The organism triggers the production of antibodies. Those antibodies will later protect the body if it encounters the same organism. And the reason cowpox vaccination works for smallpox is that the cowpox virus is closely related to that for smallpox. If a cowpox virus is injected, it will provoke antibodies that cross-react with the smallpox virus.

The twentieth century has seen fantastic vaccine developments. They are all based on the vaccination principles laid down by the Chinese, Arabs, Jenner, and

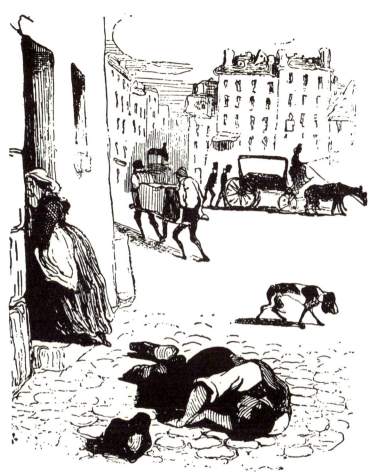

"Souvenirs of the Cholera," an etching by Honoré Daumier. Before vaccination and sanitary measures against this terrible disease were developed, epidemics of it killed people in great numbers. In 1853 and 1854, 150,000 people in France died of it, and in that same decade about 4000 were victims of it in New York City alone. The organism, Vibrio comma, causes severe vomiting and diarrhea; the loss of water from the tissues in this way is the principal cause of death.

Pasteur. Vaccines made from weakened or dead germs, or from closely related germs, are now available for 20 diseases. These include smallpox, rabies, cholera, typhoid, whooping cough, diphtheria, scarlet fever, staph infection, tetanus, typhus, Rocky Mountain spotted fever, influenza, mumps, tuberculosis, yellow fever, polio, adenovirus infection, measles, mumps, and German measles. And the diseases for which vaccines are available are increasing almost every year now. Those looming large are strep throat, hepatitis, meningitis, pneumococcal pneumonia, and syphilis. Each new vaccine should prove of immense value to millions of people.

Our century has also seen fantastic progress in understanding infectious diseases; that is, scientists now know which germs cause which ones. They know what kind of immunity certain germs evoke. And they know why some people are more susceptible to certain ailments.

Scientists know that a number of infectious diseases are caused by bacteria—small primitive cells formerly considered plants but now classified as monerans. The diseases include cholera, tetanus, tuberculosis, pneumococcal pneumonia, and others. All these diseases caused thousands of deaths among Americans until vaccines or effective drugs were developed against them.

The body's main defenses against bacterial infections appear to be antibodies. The B cells "recognize" particular bacteria, then dispatch the right antibodies to fight them. But macrophages also appear to play an important role in the defense against bacteria.

Tuberculosis bacteria, for instance, are small enough to skip around immune defenses in a person's nose and throat; thus they get into the lungs. There they make copies of themselves, then travel into the lymph nodes and bloodstream. Now the macrophages try to destroy the bacteria. Whether they do so or not will probably determine whether the person gets tuberculosis. If a person's macrophages conquer tuberculosis bacteria, they never "forget" it—one will get a positive reaction on a tuberculin skin test. There are some 15 million Americans whose macrophages have thus shown that they once conquered tuberculosis bacteria. Pneumococcal pneumonia is another disease in which macrophages are important. But the bacteria that cause this disease are coated with sugar capsules. This makes it hard for macrophages to destroy them.

The Strange Viruses

A number of infectious diseases are also caused by viruses. These are extremely small cores of genetic material surrounded by proteins. Most scientists no longer consider them to be living things. Serious diseases caused by viruses include meningitis, hepatitis, and polio. Less serious viral diseases include the common cold, flu, diarrhea, fever blisters, and warts. Vaccines are available against a number of viral diseases. But drugs that are effective against viruses are still largely unavailable.

The main immune defenses against viruses appear to

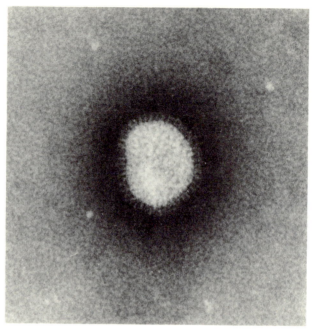

This is a Type A influenza virus, photographed by an electron microscope. As reproduced here, it has been magnified about 188,000 times. Flu of various types represents only one of many ailments and serious diseases caused by viruses.

be antibodies. For instance, IgGs in the body generally and IgAs in the nose and throat are critical fighters against the common cold. But macrophages also engage in the fighting. And so do T cells, certainly more than in the fight against bacteria. There are still other proteins that play an important role in the fight against viruses. These proteins together are called interferon.

Interferon is different from the major immune forces in several respects. It is made by the cells that are attacked by viruses. So it tends to protect these cells from within. And the immune defenses protect them from without.

Soviet immunologists found that a certain chemical that blocks interferon also blocks T cells and antibodies. This suggests that T cells, antibodies, and interferon probably interact in protecting cells from viruses. But how they interact is still a mystery.

Infectious diseases can be caused by still other agents that are in between bacteria and viruses. For instance, Rocky Mountain spotted fever was a dread disease among settlers of Montana toward the latter part of the nineteenth century. Today the cause of the disease is known: small rod-shaped organisms known as rickettsiae. Exactly how immune fighters handle rickettsiae needs more exploration.

And some infectious diseases are caused by organisms called parasites. Like viruses, they depend on host cells for survival. They are in some cases larger than bacteria and viruses. Toxoplasmosis is one infectious disease that is caused by a minute parasite, the toxoplasma. The disease is usually mild. But if a pregnant woman gets it, there is a good chance that the parasite will damage the brain of her unborn baby. Fungi—plant parasites—cause athlete's foot. And there is a terrible ailment called Chagas' disease that is triggered by a parasitic protozoan, or one-celled animal, called a trypanosome.

It causes heart damage, swellings, running sores, and sometimes idiocy.

Both T cells and antibodies play major roles in fighting off parasites. If certain parasitic worms attack the body, for instance, T cells seem to "recognize" them. Then the T cells probably alert the B cells, and these make antibodies against the worms, especially IgE antibodies. In Chagas' disease, T cells try to kill the invading parasite. But during the battle they automatically destroy heart tissue and end up hurting the body rather than helping it.

A mother's antibodies try to protect her unborn baby from the parasites that cause toxoplasmosis. However, these antibodies usually don't reach the baby's brain, where they are especially needed. The reason is that the cells that line the brain's capillaries (the smallest blood vessels) and the glial cells (which form a wall around these capillaries and the brain's nerve cells) will not let them through.

Kuru

There is the mysterious category of infectious enemies known as slow viruses. They are undoubtedly the most fascinating of the enemies that cause infectious diseases. And they nearly always lead to death.

During the 1950s, a medical officer in Australia, Victor Zigas, discovered that thousands of persons living in New Guinea suffered from a strange brain disease. They trembled. They became stiff. They swayed like

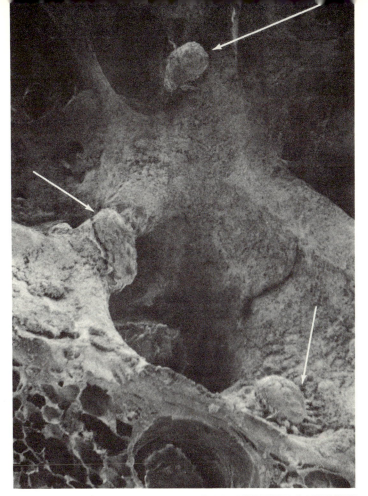

NATIONAL INSTITUTES OF HEALTH

Parasites of all kinds play a part in causing various ailments. In this electron-microscope picture the arrows point to three lung mites—very small animals related to spiders—in a monkey's lung wall. The lung's reaction is to thicken locally and become granular. The investigators also found an immune response: the mites' legs and body surfaces became coated with inflammatory cells that slowed their movements. Mites, to which we usually pay little attention, are more numerous than any other arachnids, or spider-like animals.

drunkards. They passed into comas and died. The New Guinea highlanders called the disease kuru. "Kuru" means "fear of trembling." Dr. Zigas reported the disease to the Australian authorities. After that, he and D. Carlton Gajdusek of the National Institutes of Health published scientific papers on kuru. Dr. Gajdusek then devoted several years to studying the pathology and transmission of kuru.

In 1959, Dr. William Hadlow, an American veterinarian, was working in England. He heard about kuru. He noted a similarity between the brain damage caused by kuru and that inflicted by scrapie. Scrapie is a fatal brain disease of sheep. More and more scientists thought that scrapie was caused by a slow-acting infectious agent, probably a virus. Dr. Hadlow thought kuru might also be induced by a so-called slow virus. He sent an account of his observations to the British medical journal *Lancet*.

Dr. Gajdusek read Dr. Hadlow's write-up in *Lancet*. He then visited scientists who were working on scrapie. With the help of the NIH, he set up research to look into human diseases that might be caused by slow viruses. In 1967, Dr. Gajdusek and a colleague, Clarence Gibbs, Jr., reported that the material from kuru victims infected monkeys. And it took monkeys three years to get kuru. It also takes lab animals months or several years to come down with scrapie. So Drs. Gajdusek and Gibbs concluded that kuru is also triggered by a slow virus.

Their evidence was bolstered by the virtual disappearance of kuru among the New Guinea highlanders by the late 1960s. The highlanders had been advised to give up their cannibalistic rite of eating brain tissue from dead relatives. Apparently a kuru virus was passed from the brain tissue into their own bodies. Drs. Gajdusek and Gibbs have since shown that this brain tissue teemed with infectious agents.

The kuru drama is remarkable for several reasons. It is the first strong evidence for a slow-virus disease in people. Since then, slow viruses have also appeared to be the causes of some other slowly developing, lethal human diseases. One of these diseases is multiple sclerosis. This disease destroys the nervous system and leads to loss of coordination and finally paralysis. It is especially tragic because it usually strikes persons under the age of 20.

What are slow viruses, then? Are they special kinds of viruses that are slow to kill? Or are they conventional viruses that, for some reason, become killers? The conventional measles virus has been found in the brains of multiple-sclerosis victims. This fact suggests that the latter theory may be right. On the other hand, slow-virus diseases may consist of a person's slow immune response to conventional viruses.

Scientists have found that kuru victims do not make immune defenses against kuru. T cells from multiple-sclerosis victims were exposed to measles virus. The T cells responded poorly to the virus. On the other hand, slow-virus victims can make some immune responses. Antibodies to measles virus have been found in the blood of persons with multiple sclerosis. Swedish immunologists believe that multiple sclerosis consists of a chronic measles infection. The immune system attacks the measles virus. Then the virus gets the upper hand again.

So it's quite possible that slow-virus diseases are the result of inadequate immune defenses. Once immunologists better understand immune reactions in slow-virus patients, they will probably get at the causes of these diseases.

Certain people, then, may be more susceptible to slow-virus diseases than others are. This is because their immune armies are not as strong as they should be. In fact, immunologists now know that people can vary remarkably in their susceptibility to all kinds of infectious diseases.

Warts, for instance, usually attack adolescents or young adults. This age association suggests that adolescents or young adults probably have some immune deficiency that makes them susceptible to warts. It is probably some antibody deficiency. During 1973, Finnish investigators studied 182 persons with warts. They found that only half the persons had antibodies against warts in their blood. The longer the persons had warts, the fewer antibodies they had. And the antibodies that appeared to be especially important against warts were of the IgE type.

Immunologists also believe that persons who succumb to tuberculosis have immune systems that are especially vulnerable to that disease. And some young persons seem to be more open to infectious mononucleosis, or "mono." This is also jokingly referred to as the kissing disease; the reason is that it is spread by the mouth and throat. A virus known as the herpes virus is believed to cause mono. Those who lack antibodies to this particular virus are known to be more susceptible to the disease.

Fever blisters are definitely known to be caused by a herpes virus. Scientists have found that those persons who get fever blisters have sluggish T cells against the virus. And persons who get fever blisters tend to get them again and again.

In fact, each of us probably has different immune defenses against each infectious disease. Alice may have greater immune protection against measles than her friend Tim has. But Tim may have greater protection against mono than Alice has. And Alice's friend Laura may have even greater protection against measles than Alice has—but Laura may be more susceptible to fever blisters than Alice. Immunologists hope they will someday know much more about which persons are susceptible to which infectious diseases. Then each of us can make a point of staying well away from cases of those diseases that our immune forces can't handle.

Meanwhile immunologists and infectious-disease experts have a more pressing challenge: bringing immunology and infectious-disease advances to persons in developing countries. Infectious diseases still make millions of Americans sick, but they don't cause deaths among Americans the way they used to. However, infectious diseases are still the main cause of death among peoples in the developing countries.

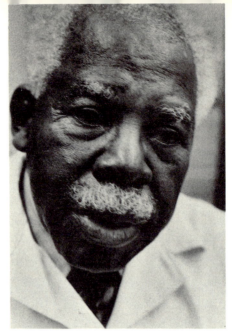

Dr. Hildrus Poindexter of Howard University worked his way from the rural South to attend high school, college, and ultimately Harvard Medical School, struggling with racial prejudice all the way. Today he is one of the nation's experts on infectious-disease problems in the developing countries, especially Africa. He is a warm and compassionate man who can well serve as a stimulus to young people of all races who want to enter the world of medicine.

Dr. Hildrus Poindexter is a research physician with Howard University in Washington, D.C. He is one of America's authorities on infectious diseases in the developing countries. He tells us that the major diseases facing peoples in Africa, Asia, and South America are tropical ailments caused by parasites. These diseases are mostly limited to the tropics because that is where the parasites thrive. Such diseases include malaria, schistosomiasis, hookworm, and river blindness.

The Burden of the Tropical Diseases

Let's take a quick look at what tropical diseases mean to persons in the developing countries. More than one billion people—an astounding number—are threatened by malaria every day of their lives. In Africa alone, malaria takes the lives of more than one million children each year. And even if youngsters survive malaria, the parasite isn't driven from their blood. As a result, they do not have the mental and physical energy that they need to learn, work, and enjoy life.

In the African country of Sierra Leone, many children dive into creeks for diamonds and gold. This is the kind of pastime that American children dream about. But nearly half the children who dive in Sierra Leone pay a severe penalty for their fun. They get schistosomiasis. This disease will not kill them. But it does something just as cruel—it saps their mental and physical energy, probably for the rest of their lives.

Hookworms, about half an inch in length, get into the intestines and feed on their lining, sucking blood and tissue fluids. This results in anemia, lack of energy, and inadequate physical and mental development. And there is river blindness. In certain areas of central Africa and South America, all adults are blind from this disease. They depend on their children to lead them around until the children become blind too.

As if these were not enough, peoples in Africa, South America, and Asia are also prey to other infectious

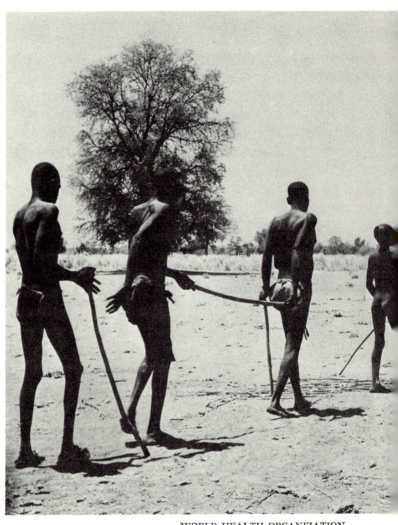

River blindness is caused by a minute worm transmitted by the bite of infected flies. These adults of Chad in Africa have become blind from the worm and have to be led about by children who can still see.

diseases, such as most Americans no longer have to worry about. Tuberculosis, diarrhea, and dysentery are high on the list.

Immunologists are studying how the immune system reacts to tropical diseases. They hope that this knowledge will help them make vaccines against them, or at least more effective drugs. They are also trying to better understand how the kind and amount of food one eats alter the immune system's ability to fight these diseases. Literally millions of persons in Asia, Africa, and South America are severely malnourished, or actually on the brink of starvation.

The investigators are finding that malnutrition indeed impairs the immune system's ability to fight tropical diseases. Persons who have too little iron, for instance, are more susceptible to malaria. B and T cells seem to need lots of iron to be robust enough for battle.

Progress is being made in getting rid of the parasites that cause tropical diseases—especially malaria. People in developing countries are learning how tropical diseases spread. In this way they can change living habits that open them to the diseases. But there is still an overwhelming amount to be done. For one thing, this means seeing that they get enough food. The World Food Conference held in Rome, Italy, during 1974 was a first step in this direction. For another, it means seeing that sanitation improves; and that the life cycles of parasites are interrupted. And many more drugs and vaccines that are now available in developed countries must also be shipped to the developing countries.

Dr. Poindexter was asked if he had any wish that could be met during the next few years. "Yes," he replied. "To get rid of malaria, hookworm, and schistosomiasis."

As things now stand, people in the developed countries have profited immensely from advances in fighting infectious diseases. But there is something else that persons in these countries now have to fear more than ever. It is cancer. We will now look at this widespread and dread disease and see how the immune system interacts with it.

5. IMMUNITY: FRIEND OR FOE IN CANCER?

Cancer. The word alone brings a feeling of dread to millions of Americans—understandably, for over half a million Americans succumb to it each year. It will strike one out of every four of us sometime during our lives. And it is the second leading cause of death in the United States.

Cancer is nothing new in the history of humanity. People have died from it down through the centuries, from King Herod of Judea through Napoleon and up to the outstanding ecologist Rachel Carson. The reason that cancer looks so impressive now is that infectious diseases have been largely conquered in the United States and in other developed countries. So today cancer and heart disease have moved up as the major causes of death.

What is cancer? Usually cells divide and increase in number in orderly fashion. When enough of them fill up a space, they stop multiplying. But cancer cells don't do this. They multiply wildly, as if they were trying to take over and blot out the entire body. As they substitute for the body's normal cells, the body becomes diseased, and this disease often leads to death.

One of America's bright young cancer scientists is Howard M. Temin of the University of Wisconsin. Dr. Temin describes cancer this way: "Cancer is a kind of violence, a disease where a part of the body wars on the rest after slipping from the normal controls of orderly growth and development."

What makes cancer cells grow and multiply wildly? This is one of the biggest questions of twentieth-century medical science. Three environmental factors loom large as causes: radiation, chemicals, and viruses. Many Japanese, for example, got cancer from the radiation given off by the atomic bomb dropped on Hiroshima in World War II. A number of chemical plant workers have gotten cancer because they were exposed to cancer-causing chemicals on the job. And while viruses have not yet been shown to trigger human cancers, they have been shown to spark certain animal cancers.

Radiation, chemicals, and viruses do not appear to be sufficient in themselves to cause cancer, though. The time and extent of exposure to these environmental factors appears to be crucial. For example, a person can have X-rays taken of his chest without their giving him cancer. One other thing appears to determine whether radiation, chemicals, and viruses will spark cancer in people or animals. This is the status of their immune systems. The more robust the immune system is, the greater are one's chances that it will wipe out newly formed cancer cells before they have a chance to get established, become tumors and eventually take over the body.

"Every Week We May Get Cancer"

There is ample evidence that the immune system plays such a protective role. Individuals who have various defects in their immune systems appear to be more susceptible to cancer than are other persons. Patients with lung cancer have lower levels of T cells than do healthy persons. Women with breast cancer show immune defects. Children with cancer show various levels of lymphocytes. Those with more lymphocytes were more successful in fighting off the disease than the ones with fewer lymphocytes. People who receive drugs that suppress immunity are especially vulnerable. Cancer tends to strike older people, whose immune systems have lost strength.

"Every week we may get cancer. And every week we may reject it," declares Robert A. Good. Dr. Good heads the renowned Sloan-Kettering Institute in New York City. He is also one of the great pioneers in twentieth-century immunology. Sound immune systems, then, probably explain why more of us do not come down with cancer.

If this is true, which immune fighters protect us from cancer? Lymphocytes, especially T cells, seem to hold the major position, according to Dr. Bernard Amos, a dynamic immunologist at Duke University in North Carolina. He performed experiments that dramatically illustrate this role. He injected cancer cells into the abdomen of a laboratory animal. The cells multiplied; ten days later there were a billion of them. Then something happened, Dr. Amos recalls, that was "explosive." Several million lymphocytes invaded the abdomen and wiped out the billion cancer cells in one day. These results, he concludes, "are a first-class measure of the power of the immune system."

Dr. Amos and his team are now trying to see why lymphocytes, specifically T cells, are able to "recognize" cancer cells. They also want to know why they can fight them off so successfully.

Macrophages also appear to be important. T cells give off a chemical called MIF, for "migration inhibition factor." MIF helps herd macrophages together, which helps in attacking cancer cells. Macrophages are able to distinguish between cancer cells and normal cells. Complement proteins, and perhaps interferon as well, may also assist in the battle against cancer.

Antibodies seem to help T cells in the struggle. A husband-wife team at the University of Washington, Karl and Ingegerd Hellström, took T cells from a patient with a tumor. They put the T cells with tumor cells taken from the patient. Then they took antibodies from the patient and put them with the patient's tumor cells.

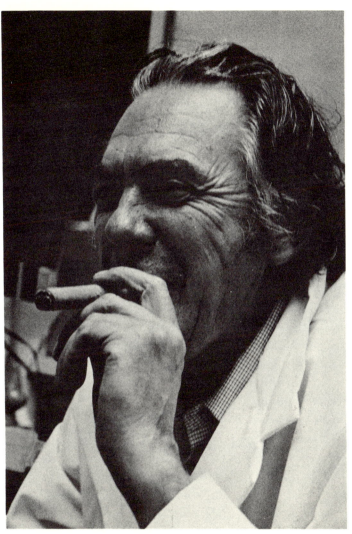

Dr. Bernard Amos, an energetic man with a keen sense of humor, is working on several different aspects of immunity research, notably the genetics behind the immune system and immune defenses against cancer.

The antibodies helped the T cells kill the tumor cells more swiftly than the T cells could do alone. But without the T cells, the antibodies were powerless.

There is disturbing evidence, however, that antibodies may sometimes be a traitor to the body in the fight. This evidence comes from the laboratory of the Hellströms; and other scientists are getting similar results. Antibodies usually bind themselves to complement, and together they attack cancer cells. But if complement isn't present, the antibodies tend to bind themselves to protein or sugar molecules on the cancer cells. And when this happens, antibody-antigen complexes are formed. These complexes seem to help protect cancer rather than destroy it.

Dr. Kathleen Ambrose of the Oak Ridge National Laboratory in Tennessee offers another explanation. She suggests that antibodies try to defend the body against cancer but if there are too many cancer antigens to cope with, the antibodies link up with the antigens. This linking up "confuses" T cells. The T cells fail to attack the cancer cells and thus cancer gets an upper hand.

There is also some evidence that cancer cells have weapons of their own to fend off the immune fighters. For instance, they give off a chemical that keeps macrophages from engulfing them. The chemical may also keep T cells and complement from striking them down.

On the whole, the immune system seems to fight off cancer actively rather than merely try to protect it. A number of immunologists are convinced that this is indeed the case, so they are trying to alter the immune systems of cancer patients.

A Vaccine for Cancer?

Dr. Georges Mathé of the Paul-Brousse Hospital outside of Paris is an energetic and compassionate doctor. Back in 1964 he did something that had never been done before. He gave Bacillus Calmette-Guérin (BCG), a tuberculosis vaccine made of tuberculosis bacteria, to some children dying from leukemia. This disease is cancer of the white blood cells. Animal studies had led him to believe that the vaccine might prime the children's immune systems against cancer.

His results were remarkable. Some of his young patients are still alive today, 10 years later. Children with leukemia rarely live beyond five years. Dr. Mathé's success set the stage for a new approach: improving the immune status of cancer patients.

Since then he has given BCG to other cancer patients, with ample success. So have some other researchers. They include Drs. Good and his colleagues at the Sloan-Kettering Institute, Joseph E. Sokal of the Roswell Park Memorial Institute in Buffalo, N.Y., and Saul Rosenberg of the Stanford University School of Medicine in San Francisco. BCG can extend the lives of patients with leukemia, skin cancer, and cancer of the lymph tissues.

The vaccine seems to be most effective when combined with other forms of therapy. Dr. Donald Morton of the University of California at Los Angeles has been

using surgery to cut out big tumors in patients. He then
gives patients BCG to clean up any cancer cells that
surgery didn't get.

How BCG primes the immunity of cancer patients
isn't clear. It seems to activate macrophages and increase the alertness of lymphocytes. But it probably
doesn't prime immune fighters specifically against cancer cells. After all, the vaccine is made of tuberculosis
bacteria. If it is going to be specific, it is going to spark
immunity geared specifically to tuberculosis bacteria.

Still other nonspecific immune primers are being tried
against cancer. They include oil emulsions and various
drugs. These primers usually act on T cells. But they
are known to act also on B cells and macrophages.

In theory, an injection of cancer cells should work
better than BCG in priming the immunity of cancer
patients. And, in fact, some investigators are trying
such injections. Dr. Ludwik Gross, of the Veterans
Administration Hospital in the Bronx, New York City,
tried inducing specific immunity against leukemia in
guinea pigs. He inoculated them with very small doses
of leukemia cells. In about half the animals the leukemia
lessened or disappeared. These are gratifying results.
A spontaneous recovery from leukemia has never been
shown in people, and only rarely in animals.

Dr. J. U. Gutterman of the University of Texas has
found that cancer patients can be immunized with an
animal cancer virus. When they are, it increases their
immunity. But whether this increase will conquer their

cancers remains to be tested. If it does, it will also be evidence for a viral cause for human cancer.

Dr. Morton is giving some cancer patients tumor cell injections plus BCG. He expects the tumor cell injections to be more effective than BCG. The reason, he says, is that the tumor cells should provoke a specific immune reaction against cancer.

Still another form of immunotherapy for cancer looks promising. This is transfer factor, a chemical extracted from the lymphocytes of a person who has overcome cancer. The precise nature of this chemical is not known, but it apparently contains some form of heightened immunity against the disease. Transfer factor has been injected into some patients and helped them resist their cancers. It was used to boost the immunity of 12-year-old Ted Kennedy, Jr., the son of Senator Edward Kennedy. Ted, Jr. lost a leg to cartilage cancer.

Interferon is also being given to cancer patients. The hope is to help protect them from infectious diseases. Cancer patients often get diseases such as pneumonia because they take drugs that suppress their immune systems. Whether interferon helps or hurts tumors isn't known.

Ohio State University scientists are trying to transfer cancer immunity from animals to cancer patients. First they extracted RNA molecules from the lymphocytes of animals that had overcome cancer. RNA is the translator of genetic information in the cell. They assumed that the RNA from the lymphocytes contained genetic

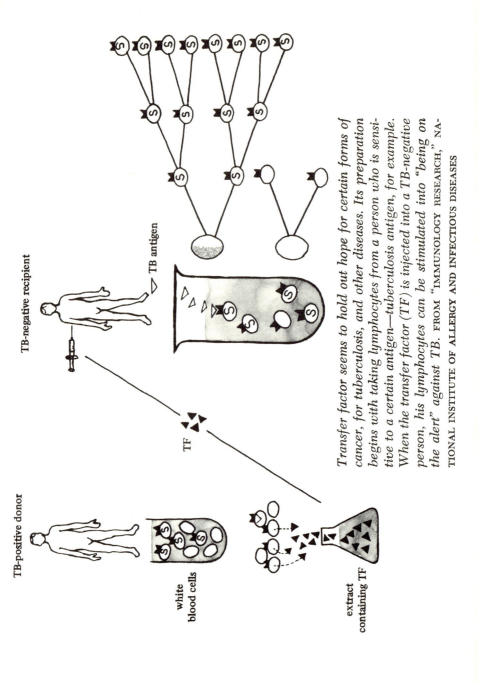

TB-positive donor

white blood cells

extract containing TF

TB-negative recipient

TB antigen

TF

Transfer factor seems to hold out hope for certain forms of cancer, for tuberculosis, and other diseases. Its preparation begins with taking lymphocytes from a person who is sensitive to a certain antigen—tuberculosis antigen, for example. When the transfer factor (TF) is injected into a TB-negative person, his lymphocytes can be stimulated into "being on the alert" against TB. FROM "IMMUNOLOGY RESEARCH," NATIONAL INSTITUTE OF ALLERGY AND INFECTIOUS DISEASES material that coded for immunity. They exposed white blood cells from cancer patients to the RNA. The RNA enabled the white cells to attack tumors under test-tube conditions. Their aim now is to take such white cells, with souped-up immunity, and inject them into cancer patients.

Immunologists would also like to use immunotherapy on patients with brain tumors. These are nearly always fatal, partly because the immune fighters of the body seem to have trouble getting into the brain.

All these attempts at immunotherapy are intriguing. And promising. But as Dr. Morton puts it, they are still "in the horse and buggy days." In other words, they don't always mean a cancer cure. Far from it. In some instances they have even made things worse—BCG, for instance, has been known to stimulate cancer in patients rather than suppress it. And it may well be because BCG stimulates antibodies, and these protect cancer rather than fight it.

Will immunotherapy of cancer turn out to be a big boon? Only time will tell. Meanwhile investigators are also looking into the value of using immunological techniques to detect cancer early in patients.

A Fetal Protein for Diagnosis

During the past decade, researchers have found that a protein normally present in the fetus pops up in children or adults with cancer. They named this protein the carcinoembryonic antigen (CEA). At first they thought it was specific for persons with cancer of the colon. Then they found that patients with other kinds of cancer have CEA as well. After that they found that healthy persons have the protein too. Finally they discovered that persons with cancer have CEA in their blood in greater amounts than do healthy persons.

A number of research groups in the United States obtained these findings. One was at the Hoffman-La-Roche Pharmaceutical Company in New Jersey. This firm obtained approval from the U. S. Food and Drug Administration to test 10,000 persons for levels of CEA in their blood. Some of the persons were known to have cancer. Some were suspected of having cancer. Still others were thought not to have cancer. CEA was found in the blood of most, but not all, of the subjects. What was significant was the amount. If a person had a very small amount of CEA, he possibly had cancer. If a person had a little more, he most likely had cancer. And if a person had much more, he almost surely had cancer.

So this discovery opened up the possibility of using CEA as a tool to figure out who has cancer. And, it was hoped, the disease could be diagnosed before it was very far advanced.

But the value of CEA as a diagnostic tool is not yet certain. First some questions have to be answered. For example, is CEA specific for certain kinds of cancers but not for others? The persons Hoffman-LaRoche tested turned out to have all kinds of cancers. CEA tests also raise an ethical question. What is the point of diagnosing cancer early if patients cannot be treated early because of uncertainty as to the type they have? Many of the patients indicated by the tests to have cancer did not develop specific tumors until months later. By the time a clinician knew exactly what kinds of cancer they had it was often too late to treat them effectively. Only when CEA assays are linked with specific cancers will early diagnosis make early treatment possible.

A Chicago doctor has also developed an immunological test that should help in the early diagnosis of cancer. The test determines blood-group antigens in samples of tissues. These are the antigens on red blood cells that differ from one person to another. They determine whether a person with a particular kind of blood antigen can receive a blood transfusion from a person with another kind. The doctor found that these antigens are lost when cancer develops. He studied nearly a thousand patients. He found that when the antigens were absent, cancer was present. And when the antigens were present, cancer was less likely.

There are active searches under way for cancer vaccines. A vaccine against breast cancer in mice has been developed by New Jersey researchers. It consists of killed mouse breast-tumor virus. A single dose seems to prime a mouse's cellular immunity and protect it against cancer. Mouse breast cancer and human breast cancer are a lot alike; they may be caused by related viruses. So it may be possible to use the mouse-tumor virus to make a vaccine against human breast cancer.

Dr. André Nahmias, professor of pediatrics and head

of a viral-cancer study team at the Emory University School of Medicine, was among the first scientists in the 1960s to announce an apparent link between herpes simplex virus infections and cancer of the uterus in women. Dr. Nahmias and his team are attempting to develop a vaccine from this virus. They hope that eventually the vaccine can be used to protect women against cancer of the uterus.

Probably the most hopeful cancer vaccine work is being carried out by German scientists. They managed to do what had never been done before. They vaccinated monkeys against a kind of cancer caused by a herpes virus. Monkeys are closely related to humans, so the researchers hope that a similar vaccine might work for people. If it does work, it will probably be used for human cancer caused by a herpes virus, such as mostly strikes African children.

There is little doubt that the future will bring a better understanding of cancer. Whatever advances are made, immunity will surely be closely linked with them. Dr. Frank J. Rauscher, Jr., president of the National Cancer Institute, believes that immunology is one of the brightest long-range hopes in the cancer research field.

6. IMMUNE DEFENSES TURN TRAITOR

Lisa M. was young, bright, and bubbly. She had been healthy almost all of her 14 years. That is, until a humid day in August when a wasp stung her on the arm. The sting was painful but felt no worse than it had once before. Then something different happened. Something swift, ominous, terrible.

Twenty minutes after the bite, Lisa started to feel funny. She gasped for breath. She couldn't think clearly. She turned a sickish, bluish color. She fell down while walking to her bedroom. Her father rushed her to the hospital. It was 11 in the morning.

She was put in a hospital bed. Perspiration ran down her cheeks. White froth foamed from her lips. Her lungs tightened to the point of suffocation. The doctors listened for her heartbeats. They heard only the faintest whisper. They gave her oxygen and drugs. She became violently sick to her stomach.

By 2:30 in the afternoon she felt much better. Her heartbeats were stronger. The doctors detected antibodies to the poison of wasps in her bloodstream. They knew then what had happened to her. She had experienced a violent reaction to wasp toxin. She experienced this reaction even though she had not reacted violently the first time she was stung.

Thanks to excellent and prompt medical care, Lisa recovered. But not all victims of similar reactions are so lucky. Some of them die.

A strong reaction like this is called anaphylaxis. What it is, really, is one example of how the body's immune system can turn traitor. The immune fighters, for mysterious reasons, begin working against the body. Such reactions also include common allergies, asthma, and the autoimmune diseases. When antibodies try to protect cancer, they too act as turncoats.

Allergies: Nuisances and Killers

An allergy is an adverse immunologic reaction against any number of substances. These substances include fish, beef, milk, eggs, berries, nuts, chocolate, cereals, and some other foods. They include smoke, dust from toys, pillows, drapes. They include hairs from dogs and cats. And they include pollen from ragweed, sagebrush, tumbleweed, and many other plants. Flaming red sumac looks beautiful in the fall and poison ivy curling up trees is a graceful summer decoration. But both kinds of plants can spell allergy anguish. Various dyes and household chemicals, and even light, heat, and cold can arouse allergic reactions.

Many people who live in San Francisco are rose-growers. They usually prune their roses in January. One January, many of these gardeners turned up at a San Francisco hospital. They all had allergic symptoms. A physician at the hospital was intrigued by their common condition and wanted to find out why they all had similar symptoms. He discovered that most of the gardeners had planted their roses near juniper bushes. When they cut back their roses, they reacted adversely to the pollen given off by the juniper bushes.

If a person is allergic to a substance, he reacts to it whenever he comes into contact with it. Allergy victims may announce their presence with sneezes, wheezes, teary eyes, runny noses, itching and skin rashes, nausea, breathing difficulty, and other troubles. Allergic youngsters often rub their noses upward in a so-called allergic salute. The salute indicates that their noses are blocked and itchy. Allergies are common. One American out of six—some 36 million of us—is allergic to something or other.

Anaphylaxis is also an allergy. But it is far more abrupt and violent than conventional allergies. It can kill. Conventional allergies rarely do so. They are just a pain to live with.

When a person is allergic to a particular substance, this antigenic substance is called an allergen. The allergen combines with those B cells in lung, nose, and throat that make IgE antibodies. The allergen also com-

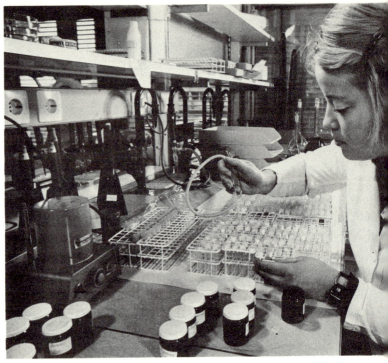

SWEDISH INTERNATIONAL PRESS BUREAU

Blood samples from allergic patients being analyzed in a Swedish laboratory. An allergen combines with those B cells in the blood that make IgE antibodies.

bines with certain T cells. The B cells, with the help of the T cells, make IgEs to the allergen.

The IgEs then hook up with the allergen. They also plug into mast cells and white cells. Once IgEs and these cells hook up, the cells pour out loads of histamine. The histamine is what makes allergy victims feel teary and awful.

Not all allergic reactions involve IgEs, though. Allergies to poison ivy and certain drugs involve lymphocytes in the spleen, lymph nodes, and blood. These lymphocytes give off migration inhibition factor. MIF seems to serve as a mediator—a transmitter and controller—for the allergic responses.

Antibodies besides IgE also appear to participate in some allergic reactions. They include IgM, IgG and IgA. Complement and macrophages seem to get in on the treasonous acts too.

On the whole, though, IgEs appear to be the major culprits in allergies. People who are allergic tend to have more IgEs in their bloodstreams than do nonallergic persons. This high level of IgE is probably under genetic control.

So IgEs are usually blamed for allergies. But European immunologist Dr. George M. Halpern points out that they probably do some good for the body as well. IgEs seem to be the first class of antibody produced during a normal, healthy immune response. Then the big fighters —IgM, IgG, IgA, and complement—get into the battle. "Too often," Dr. Halpern declared in a recent issue of the *Annals of Allergy*, "we fail to see the patrol of scouts which at 6 o'clock in the morning get out of their holes to explore the landscape and to detect an eventual enemy behind the lines."

Asthma is a disease of the lungs. Some nine million Americans have it. A third of all asthma victims are adolescents and teenagers. It's hard to forget the sight of an asthma victim having an attack. He breathes rapidly and gasps for air. Spasms of coughing wrack his body. His lungs wheeze so loudly that he sounds as if he is drowning. And in a sense, he is. His lungs are so swollen with fluid that fresh air cannot get into them. Asthma kills 3,000 Americans each year.

Asthma can be triggered by allergies. First IgEs in the lungs hook up with allergens. The IgEs also make contact with mast cells. The mast cells release histamine. This chemical causes spastic contraction of smooth muscles in the lung area, practically closing down the fine tubes of the lungs. Thus stale air is shut in the lungs, and fresh air cannot get in. As a result asthma develops. Even if a victim survives the attack, IgEs and complement can lead to a second attack a few hours later.

But asthma isn't always caused by allergies. It can also be set off by viruses that cause colds or flu. And it can be triggered by emotional upsets, or by hormone changes during adolescence or other times of life. Outside factors aren't enough to set off asthma, though. There also has to be some kind of genetic predisposition toward it.

"Immunity Against Oneself"

On the whole, quite a bit is known about the immune reactions behind allergies and asthma. But the immune reactions underlying the so-called autoimmune diseases are much more mysterious. In fact, some scientists question the existence of autoimmune diseases altogether.

What is sure, though, is that something is drastically wrong in these diseases. And immunity certainly seems to be an accomplice.

"Autoimmunity" means "immunity against oneself." In those diseases suspected of being autoimmune, certain components of the immune system appear to attack specific tissues or organs. In animals, for instance, there is a disease called allergic encephalomyelitis. This disease can be produced in animals by injecting them with a protein taken from their own nervous systems. One wouldn't expect the animals' immune systems to view this protein as foreign. But they do. T cells invade the animals' nerves. And when this happens, the animals become paralyzed and die. What's more, if these T cells are injected into other animals, those animals also come down with the disease. So it looks as if allergic encephalomyelitis is truly an autoimmune disease. And the T cells are the traitors. In fact, antibodies seem to try to protect the body against the traitors. They seem to bind to the protein the T cells attack. In this way the T cells cannot attack the protein.

There is a human disease that is somewhat like allergic encephalomyelitis. It is called postvaccinal encephalomyelitis. It is a rare complication that results only once in a while in persons who have been vaccinated against rabies. Very possibly this disease is also an autoimmune disease.

Some immunologists believe that multiple sclerosis is also autoimmune. Multiple sclerosis is a disease of the fatty sheaths that surround nerves. As mentioned before, it destroys the body slowly yet surely. These investigators thought that it might be triggered by the body's immune system attacking protein in the sheaths. They tested this theory. Sure enough, they found what they were looking for.

There is a disease that strikes especially women in their twenties. It is called lupus erythematosus. It consists of inflammation of tissues in the body or of scaly patches on the skin of the nose, scalp, or the area behind the ears. The disease can also infect the kidneys and even lead to death. But it is usually less severe than that and comes and goes over a period of years. It appears to be an autoimmune ailment. Its sufferers have antibodies that seem to react with protein in their skin. The antibodies combine with the protein. However, the complexes, or combinations, produced in this way may serve a protective function. They may keep protein in the skin from escaping into the bloodstream to combine with antibody there. Complexes in the blood would probably be harmful. So the antibodies do not seem to be the real traitors in this disease. Rather, the traitors appear to be T cells. And macrophages too. Inflammatory cells in the skin of lupus victims usually consist of T cells and macrophages.

Another disease that usually strikes young adult women is myasthenia gravis. This causes muscular weakness. Sometimes it leads swiftly to death. It appears to be autoimmune in nature. Antibodies have been found directed against muscle tissue in the victims. The victims also have abnormal thymuses. Their T cells have also been found to react with other kinds of white blood cells.

Adult rheumatoid arthritis too may be autoimmune. It consists of pain, stiffness, and inflammation of the joints. These symptoms come and go. Rheumatoid arthritis inflicts some eight million Americans and actually cripples many of them.

Virtually all the immune fighters seem to conspire against the body in rheumatoid arthritis. IgEs are suspected of triggering inflammation. So are IgGs. IgGs attack each other rather than invaders. When they attack each other, they form rheumatoid complexes. Such complexes have been found in the blood and joint fluids of 70 per cent of the victims. Macrophages appear to contribute to the inflammation as well. They release enzymes that may interact with the rheumatoid complexes and cause tissue damage.

Complement appears to lead to the destruction of bone. T cells also appear to be traitors, "conspiring" with B cells. In one experiment, lymphocytes were taken from rats with arthritis. The lymphocytes were injected into healthy rats. The rats came down with arthritis.

Children can also get rheumatoid arthritis. In fact, it strikes one out of every 10,000 youngsters. However, only one-fifth of these individuals have rheumatoid complexes. They also all have lots of antibodies directed against common viruses. So it looks as if juvenile rheumatoid arthritis is not autoimmune in nature. It is probably caused by a virus, or viruses.

A disease that causes one-third of all cases of blindness may possibly be autoimmune. A Georgetown Medical School physician removed the retinas—the light-sensitive tissues—from the eyes of healthy monkeys. He isolated certain chemicals from the retinas and injected them into other healthy monkeys. These animals became blind. It looked as if the chemicals prompted the animals' immune systems to turn against their own retinas.

As mentioned earlier, Chagas' disease seems to be triggered by a parasite. The parasite causes heart damage. But what is especially intriguing about this disease is that it seems to be a combination of infectious and autoimmune actions. A parasite crawls over its unwary victim during the night. The parasite deposits antigenic material in the victim. This material makes its way into the victim's heart. And for some unknown reason, the material provokes lymphocytes to attack the victim's heart. So it looks as if Chagas' disease is an autoimmune disease triggered by an infectious agent.

Obviously, many more questions still have to be answered about autoimmune diseases. The first is whether the diseases are really a case of immunity turning against the body. It's quite possible that they are first triggered by infectious agents. Then somehow autoimmune mixups get under way and damage the body. And whether these mixups occur could well depend on basic genetic defects in immunity. "Any time the immune system is disturbed in its basic structure," Dr. Good declares, "it can open the door to diseases that we think of as autoimmune."

New Tests for Old Troubles

Meanwhile, immunologists are making progress in the diagnosis and treatment of those diseases in which immunity turns traitor. Ever since the 1920s, allergists have given skin tests to see what substances people are allergic to. In a skin test, a tiny bit of suspect allergen is scratched into the skin of a person. If the skin turns red half an hour later, the person is allergic to that particular allergen. But there are dozens of allergens that a person might react to. So skin tests are time-consuming. And not particularly pleasant. Better diagnoses for allergies would certainly be welcome.

One that looks very promising has been designed by Swedish immunologists. A blood sample is taken from a patient. A bit of the blood is placed on various paper discs. The discs contain some 50 different allergens. If IgEs in the blood react with any of these allergens, it means that the person is allergic to them. The 50 allergens make up 90 per cent of the allergens people are usually exposed to. The results of the technique are then analyzed by computer. This method is now available in some American medical centers. If it becomes widely used, immunologists can test a great many more patients than before.

An improved diagnostic test for ragweed allergy promises to be superior to skin tests. It simply shows whether macrophages from a person attack ragweed allergen in the test tube. It is based on the discovery that macrophages from persons who are allergic to ragweed cannot take up ragweed allergens nearly as well as those from nonallergic persons. So it looks as if ragweed allergy constitutes a defect in macrophage response to ragweed.

Every year four out of every thousand Americans stung by an insect show a severe allergic reaction. It has not been possible to tell which people will react so severely. Now scientists at the National Institute of Allergy and Infectious Diseases have developed a lab test that tells sensitive persons from others. They take white cells from the person to be tested. The cells are challenged with insect allergens. If they do not release histamine, the person will not overreact to insect bites. But if they release histamine, then the person will suffer a reaction. The test has shown that those tested can vary in their reactions. Some may be allergic to honeybees only, others to honeybees plus wasps; and so on.

Treatments are also slowly improving against those diseases in which immunity turns traitor. Treatments for childhood asthma now include drugs that inhibit the release of histamine, offering protection from allergens. Immunosuppressive drugs have been added to the treatment of rheumatoid arthritis. These drugs knock out lymphocytes' ability to react, and this helps fight the disease. But it can also make patients more susceptible to infectious agents. This is because one of the body's main immune fighters has been made powerless.

California researchers have designed a more radical treatment for arthritis patients who have not been helped by drugs. A small cut is made in the patient's neck and a tube is inserted through the cut into the thoracic duct. The tube, which must stay in place for several months, drains lymph out of the patient's body. Once the lymph is removed, lymphocytes are filtered out of it. Then the lymph is returned into the patient's neck through another tube. This technique has relieved patients of their rheumatoid arthritis for six months to a year. But it is not a permanent relief. And with this treatment too there is the danger of making patients vulnerable to infectious diseases.

Draining T cells from the thoracic duct has also led to a striking improvement in patients with myasthenia gravis. But here again, improvement is not lasting, and there is a heightened danger of infections.

Allergy sufferers lose millions of dollars in work hours each year. Unfortunately the only treatment now available is time-consuming, expensive, and not always effective. It consists of weekly shots of the allergen to which a person is supposedly allergic. This treatment is called desensitization. It decreases or neutralizes the IgEs that cause the trouble.

So a more effective and economical treatment is needed. One promising approach is being explored by scientists at the Upjohn Company. They are working on ways to halt the release of histamine from mast cells.

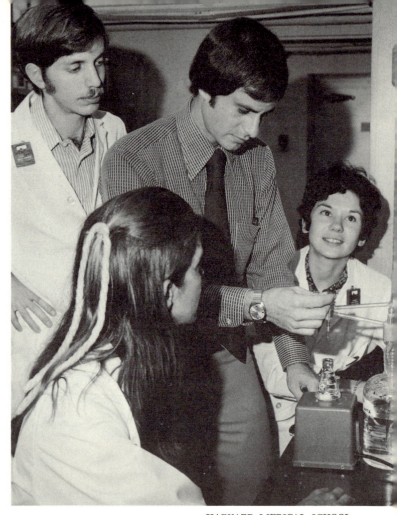

HARVARD MEDICAL SCHOOL

Much depends on teamwork in research. This group is researching new approaches to relieving allergy symptoms. Dr. Peter Newburger is standing at left, Dr. Barbara M. Osborne is seated in the foreground. Dr. David H. Katz is making a titration analysis for determining the quantity of protein nitrogen in an antigen preparation. Ms. Mary Graves, research assistant, is seated behind him. They hope to neutralize the IgEs that make trouble for allergy patients.

If they can halt the release, they think it will help sufferers from both common allergies and asthma. Immunologists at Johns Hopkins University School of Medicine are trying to inject chemically altered allergens into allergic patients. They hope that such shots will slow down IgE formation and relieve the symptoms. Dr. David H. Katz and his colleagues at Harvard Medical School are also trying to stamp out IgE production.

They found a particular chemical molecule that could switch off IgE manufacture in animals. They are now trying to hook up the "silencer" molecule to ragweed allergen (one of the worst for Americans) and other specific allergens. They hope that the silencer molecule coupled to a specific allergen might then be injected into people. Thus the chemical packet should, they hope, switch off IgE production against that particular allergen and prevent allergic responses for up to a year.

Soviet immunologists have another idea for treating allergies and perhaps even autoimmune diseases as well. This would consist of giving a chemical that knocks out interferon production. They believe that interferon might be involved in allergies and autoimmune diseases. On the other hand, interferon might be a good guy instead of a bad guy, at least in allergies. For years physicians have used bacterial vaccines to treat asthma patients. The vaccines led to some improvement, possibly by triggering the production of interferon.

7. THE CHALLENGE OF ORGAN TRANSPLANTS

It was midnight at Peter Bent Brigham Hospital in Boston. An expectant mother lay dying from kidney failure. Three of the surgeons at the hospital—Charles Hufnagel, Ernest Landsteiner, and David Hume—tried to save her life. They attached the blood vessels of a cadaver kidney to veins in the woman's arm. As a result, the kidney was partially buried under her skin. The kidney started to drain poisonous wastes from her body. Several days later, her own kidneys started secreting urine again. The cadaver kidney was removed. The woman lived.

This was the first successful temporary organ transplant. It was performed in 1945. The first successful permanent organ transplant was performed in 1954, on a patient whose kidneys had failed. Since then, 18,325 kidneys, 245 hearts, 217 livers, 35 pancreases, and 34 lungs have been permanently transplanted into patients throughout the world. All of these transplants have been performed in patients whose own organs had failed. Many of them, like the woman who received a temporary transplant, hovered between life and death. A number of these transplants, notably kidney transplants, have been successful.

Deborah P. of Chelmsford, Massachusetts, was the first youngster to undergo a kidney transplant at Children's Hospital Medical Center in Boston, in 1971. Deborah received a kidney that had been donated by her mother. "There were a lot of difficult times," Deborah's mother remembers. "But the doctors and nurses did all that we could ever ask. We both recovered very quickly. Now Debby is doing beautifully and feels fine." Deborah as a young teenager is bursting with strength and agility.

There is Kristi S. of Arlington, Virginia. Everybody thought this spunky seven-year-old was as healthy as could be—including her parents. But one day Kristi fell down at school and couldn't get up. She was taken to the hospital. It turned out that she had a kidney that had been blocked from birth. As a result, the part of the kidney that collected urine had greatly increased and had destroyed other parts of it. Kristi's doctor turned out to be no one less than Dr. Hufnagel, the organ transplant pioneer, who is now with the Georgetown Medical School in Washington, D.C. Dr. Hufnagel decided that Kristi should receive a kidney transplant. The girl is doing fine now. She is in junior high school and is active in various sports.

Not all transplant patients are as lucky as Deborah

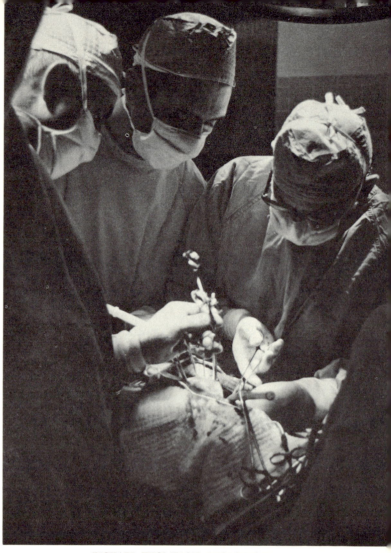

Surgeons Peter W. Conrad (left), Mario N. Gomes, and Charles A. Hufnagel do a human kidney transplant operation at Georgetown University. Although more than 18,000 kidneys have been transplanted during the past 30 years, organ transplantation still presents many problems.

and Kristi, though. And there are several reasons why. The first is surgical. The surgical techniques for kidney and heart transplantation have been pretty well worked out. But this is far from the case for liver, lung, and pancreas transplantation.

The second reason is that patients are extremely sick before they receive a new organ. For instance, those who need a new pancreas usually need a new kidney as well. Young patients usually fare better than older patients, though.

"We think children are rather favored candidates for transplants," declares Dr. Ray Levey, the surgeon who operated on Deborah. "This is because they are generally healthier than adults undergoing similar procedures." Since 1971, Dr. Levey and his colleagues at Children's Hospital Medical Center have given 45 young patients new kidneys. "We've had excellent success," Dr. Levey says. About 85 per cent of the grafts take. The children who receive the kidneys regain good health, return to school, attend gym classes and participate in sports such as horseback riding.

"Alien" Organs

There is still another reason, however, why transplants are often not successful. More often than not, the recipient's immune system views the implanted organ as foreign and tries to reject it. Physicians give transplant patients powerful drugs to blunt their immune systems. Sometimes these drugs help keep the implanted organ from being rejected. But the drugs carry risks of their own. They make patients vulnerable to infectious diseases and even cancer, because the body's immune system no longer works as it should.

During the past decade, immunologists have discovered that there are four kinds of chemical molecules on all body cells except the red blood cells. Two of the types are inherited from the mother, two from the father. The molecules are called HL-A antigens. "HL-A" comes from the words "human leukocyte antigen." "Leukocyte" is another name for a white blood cell. Thus each person has four different kinds of HL-A antigens in his body. A person's four HL-A antigens, for example, are as individual as the shape of his ears and the color of his eyes. The HL-A antigens appear to be crucial in the immunological reaction of an implanted organ.

The role of the HL-A antigens in organ rejection seems to run something like this. Let us assume that all four antigens on cells in the organ differ from the antigens in the recipient's body. Then the organ is considered definitely foreign by the recipient's immune system, and the chances of the recipient's rejecting the organ are very great. Or perhaps only two HL-As on the cells in the organ differ from antigens in the recipient's body. Then the organ is considered only somewhat foreign by the recipient's immune system; the chances of organ rejection are not so great. Or perhaps all four HL-As on the cells in the organ are identical to antigens in the recipient's body. Then the organ is not considered foreign; there is little chance of organ rejection.

Consequently, immunologists try to match donor organs and transplant recipients for HL-A antigens. In this way they hope to increase the chances of transplanted organs' being accepted.

But some 32 different HL-As have been identified so far. There are hundreds of thousands of possible combinations in the human population. It is this stupendous number of combinations that laboratories are working with as they try to match available organs with needy recipients. Fortunately the laboratories have computers to help them in the matching.

Matching a donor and recipient is not too hard if the donor is a relative. HL-A antigens are often alike or even identical among family members, just as build and facial features are. Dr. Paul I. Terasaki is a pioneer in HL-A matching at the University of California at Los Angeles. He estimates that there is a one-in-four chance of making a perfect match between brothers and sisters.

But matching an unrelated donor and recipient is far more difficult. HL-As are rarely the same among unrelated persons. Dr. Terasaki estimates that the chance of making a good match among unrelated individuals is only one in a thousand.

The importance of HL-A matching and the scientific laws that govern it are very clear to Dr. Terry Strom. He is a kidney specialist with one of the nation's largest HL-A matching laboratories, the one at Peter Bent

Brigham Hospital. Dr. Strom reports that the four-antigen match—the ideal match—gives a 95 per cent survival the first year, an 85 per cent survival the next, and so on. But a zero-antigen match does not give such a good survival rate. Dr. Terasaki also believes in the value of HL-A matching between living relative donors and recipients.

But HL-A matching does not seem to be that valuable in the transplantation of organs from unrelated persons who have just died. Dr. Norman A. Shumway of Stanford University Medical School is one of only two surgeons in the world who are doing heart transplants on a regular basis, and getting good results. To date, 69 of his patients have received new hearts. Twenty-four of them are alive as this is written. Throughout this extensive transplantation experience, Dr. Shumway and his team have found no firm link between HL-A matching and rejection.

"We match by HL-A typing. But I'm not sure it's that important," admits Dr. Marvin L. Gliedman of Montefiore Hospital in New York City. Dr. Gliedman is a pioneer in pancreas transplants.

"There is no good correlation between HL-A matches and liver transplant success," declares Dr. Thomas Starzl. Dr. Starzl was the first surgeon to do a liver transplant. He is with the Colorado General Hospital in Denver.

So HL-A matching is not the final solution to immunological rejection of transplanted organs. It's hard to match organs and recipients for all four HL-A antigens.

And even if all four antigens are matched, rejection may still occur if the organ is from a cadaver.

There may be a very good reason why HL-A matching works well when organs are from close relatives. And there may be a very good reason why it does not work well when organs are from unrelated persons. It may be that other antigens are crucial for organ acceptance.

These antigens are known to be made by genes that are closely linked to the genes that make HL-As. As a result, if organs from close relatives are well matched with those of recipients for HL-As, it is possible that the organs are also well matched for the other antigens. But if organs from unrelated persons are well matched with the HL-As of recipients, it's possible that the organs are not well matched for the other antigens. Why is this? If one person inherits a package of certain antigens, his sister or brother may well have the same package. But the chances are slim that he and a stranger will have an identical package of antigens.

There is evidence, for instance, that so-called mixed lymphocyte culture antigens—MLC antigens—may be important in transplantation. Some European investigators have reported greater success from HL-A matching in cadaver transplants than have American investigators. The reason may be that HL-As and MLCs are usually inherited as a package in homogeneous European populations. Homogeneous populations are those in which people are related to each other over many generations, as, say, in France or Germany. But it's very probable that the package of antigens has become rearranged in the more heterogeneous American population—one in which people come from many different ethnic backgrounds and are usually not related to one another. Thus, if an unrelated organ donor and an organ recipient are well matched for HL-As in Europe, they are probably also well matched for MLCs. But if an unrelated donor and recipient are well matched for HL-As in the United States, they may very well not be matched for MLCs.

So at this time, antigen matching is bringing in less than ideal results in assuring transplant success. Thus immunologists are trying to come up with a better means of countering transplant rejection. One of their major efforts is to better understand the rejection problem. "We don't know exactly how destructive action takes place," admits Dr. Anthony Monaco. Dr. Monaco is a kidney transplant surgeon with the New England Deaconess Hospital in Boston. And Dr. Hufnagel agrees: "We don't understand rejection entirely." However, tissue studies and photos taken of rejected organ tissue under the microscope suggest that rejection works this way:

Antigens from cells in the transplanted organ—say the HL-As or the MLCs—are brought by the bloodstream to the lymph nodes of the transplanted patient. There the patient's T cells become exposed to any of those antigens that are foreign to the patient's body.

The T cells are then swept by the bloodstream to the transplanted organ. The T cells attack cells in the organ that contain the foreign antigens. Macrophages and complement do too. Blood platelets and inflammatory cells also rush to the site of the invasion. The blood vessels of the organ become clogged with the invaders. The organ can no longer get nutrients from the patient's body. The organ dies.

Antibodies also participate in organ rejection. Intriguingly, however, some antibodies—or at least parts of antibodies—try to protect the transplanted organ rather than reject it. Dr. Hufnagel and his immunologist colleague Dr. Anthony Chung are trying to use this protective role of antibodies to prevent organ rejection.

The concept, which they are now testing on dogs, is this. The individual to receive an organ is immunized with lymphocytes from the organ donor. Antibodies that the individual makes against the lymphocytes are then broken down into the parts of antibodies that hook up with complement, and those that do not. The parts that hook up with complement seem to be those parts that assist in organ rejection. The other parts seem to be those that enhance organ acceptance.

These latter parts are then bubbled through the organ to be transplanted. A coat of this enhancing antibody material should help protect the organ from being rejected once it is transplanted. The organ recipient is also injected with the enhancing antibody material to further increase the chances of organ acceptance.

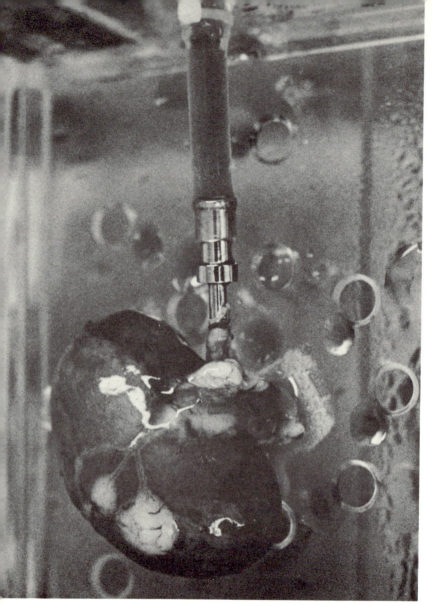

Antibody parts that do not combine with complement are bubbled through a human kidney to be transplanted; these parts help the body to accept the otherwise "alien" kidney.

Organs From the Lower Animals

Drs. Hufnagel and Chung are working on still another approach to solving the rejection problem. It would consist of using animal organs for human transplants. "Of the various approaches we are taking to the rejection problem," Dr. Hufnagel says, "this one has the greatest potential." He believes it has the greatest potential because there will never be enough human organs to supply transplantation needs. For instance, on any one day in the United States, 20,000 people have end-stage kidney disease and desperately need a transplantable kidney. But only one-tenth of these people are getting a kidney. These two investigators are now exposing different kinds of animal organs to human blood, hoping to find out which kind of organ might be the least objectionable to human immune fighters. We might eventually see the day when Dr. X asks Patient Y: "Would you like a lion's heart, sir? Or how about a chimpanzee liver?"

Drs. Hufnagel and Chung are doing still a third thing to solve the organ-rejection problem. They would like to give an organ recipient something to stop the multiplication of the T and B cells that leads to rejection. The substances they would like to use are chalones. These are chemicals that are naturally present in humans and animals; they are known to interfere with cell division. So far, the Georgetown investigators have shown that injections of chalones can delay skin-graft rejection in animals. Skin-graft rejections are similar to organ-transplant rejections; they too involve antibody and cellular immunity. Actually, grafted skin is more often rejected than are implanted organs. "We really don't know why," Dr. Hufnagel admits.

Still other doctors are trying to solve the organ-rejection problem. Dr. Monaco is injecting bone marrow from organ donors into prospective organ recipients. Bone marrow is rich in HL-A antigens. So Dr. Monaco believes that bone marrow should stimulate protective antibody action in those slated to receive organs. Thus, when individuals receive organs, their enhancing antibodies will already be primed to help protect the foreign organ. Dr. Monaco has obtained encouraging results with this approach in mice and dogs. He is now ready to try it on patients.

Dr. Monaco also looks forward to the day when HL-A antigens will have been purified in large quantities. He believes HL-As might be taken from an organ donor and injected into a would-be recipient. The would-be recipient would then make enhancing antibodies against the antigens. The enhancing antibodies would help protect the foreign organ upon implantation.

Dr. Robert J. Sharbaugh and his immunology colleagues at the Medical University of South Carolina are trying to solve the rejection problem by doing research on large animals. They are looking for the transplantation antigens in sheep that correspond to the HL-As in people. They will then coat a column with these antigens. They will insert a tube into the sheep's thoracic duct and circulate the sheep's lymph out of the tube and through the column. They hope that any lymphocytes in the lymph that usually attack transplantation antigens will stick to the antigens on the column. The lymph will then be returned into the sheep's thoracic duct. They hope that this lymph will be cleared of all lymphocytes that attack transplantation antigens. Then the sheep should be ready for an organ transplant and show no rejection problem.

"Our approach is promising," Dr. Sharbaugh asserts. "But it's tough. Few investigators are using this approach. In other words, we have little or no past experience to call on."

Still other investigators believe that a better understanding of the chemistry of transplantation antigens should lead to ways of preventing organ rejection. One of these investigators is Dr. Stanley G. Nathanson of the Albert Einstein College of Medicine in New York City. Certainly progress is being made toward this end. But so far the evidence is more mysterious than satisfying.

HL-A antigens, for instance, are now known to have some of the same chemical material that antibodies have. The antigens are also coded by genes that lie near the genes that code for various immunological activities. Such evidence suggests that transplantation antigens may have some yet unidentified immunological function. This would be bizarre since they themselves provoke immunological reactions.

It may be some years before the transplant rejection

problem is really solved. And this goes for other transplant problems as well. They include a shortage of organs for transplantation, problems of preserving organs until they can be transplanted, surgical difficulties, the physical and psychological stress of receiving a foreign organ. And then there is the great cost of organ transplants. At this time, a heart transplant at Stanford University costs $42,000. As organ transplants become less experimental and more standard treatment, their cost should come down.

Meanwhile, transplantation surgeons and immunologists have the satisfaction of extending the lives of patients a few precious months, or even years. And patients are grateful. Take the case of Ralph T. of San Francisco. A heart transplant restored this 36-year-old, self-taught organist to a vigorous life. He continues with his profession and he also skied and rode a motorcycle until he broke his back in a fall from a tree.

And then there is Richard C. of Patchogue, New York. From age 38 to 45, Richard had experienced numerous heart attacks. Surgery hadn't helped him. His body couldn't take much more. So his doctor referred him to Dr. Shumway for a heart transplant. The transplant was successful. Now, five years later, Richard works as an engineer. He swims in a pool he himself built. He works out in a private gym an hour each day. "The doctors at Stanford are wonderful," Richard says. "They gave me my life."

8. RESTORING IMMUNITY WHERE IT'S LACKING

During 1968, a five-month-old child named David C. was flown from Connecticut to the University of Minnesota. David's laboratory tests and family history had proven that he had inherited a serious immune-deficiency disease. He had no immune system because he lacked the bone marrow stem cells that make the system. Like all 12 male children on his mother's side of the family, he was marked for an early death unless something was done, and soon.

At the University of Minnesota, immunology pioneer Dr. Robert Good went to work. He and his colleagues found that David and his sister Doreen had identical transplantation antigens on their cells. This fact suggested that Doreen would be an ideal bone-marrow donor for David. Because the transplantation antigens matched, there was little chance that the bone marrow cells would reject David's body as foreign. So Dr. Good and his team took some billion bone marrow cells from Doreen's hip bone. They injected these cells into David's abdomen. They hoped that some of these cells would be the stem cells that David needed in order to develop the immune system he lacked. And they kept their fingers crossed that Doreen's bone marrow would not fatally attack David's body.

They won. A brand-new immune system sprang up in David's body. This abundant new supply of immune fighters helped David overcome his many infections. Today David is in vigorous health.

During the same year, something equally dramatic happened in a nearby state, Wisconsin. A two-year-old boy named David Z. had been diagnosed for another immune-deficiency disease. This boy had an immune system, but it had serious defects. His future looked grim. Drs. Fritz Bach of the University of Wisconsin and Mortimer Bortin of the Mount Sinai Medical Center in Milwaukee tried to save David Z.'s life.

It was obvious to the doctors that David was in a bad way. He had all kinds of infections. He was bleeding from the nose and mouth. He was fast approaching the point of no return. But in one respect David Z. was as lucky as David C. One of his two sisters, Barbara, was an ideal bone marrow donor.

David received two injections of bone marrow cells from Barbara. For two weeks it was touch and go. David's defective immune system tried to reject the implanted cells. But finally these cells won out. David's body became populated with lymphocytes made by

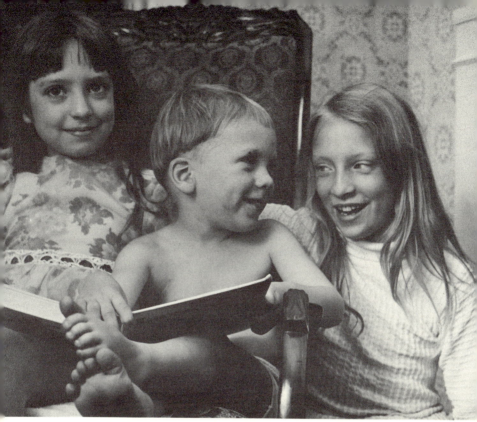

THE NATIONAL FOUNDATION—MARCH OF DIMES
David Z. with his sisters Mimi, left, and Barbara. His life was saved by Barbara's bone-marrow cells.

Barbara's contribution. With this new, healthy immune system, David's infections were overcome. Today he is a healthy child.

These case histories are gratifying because the lives of two children were saved by the heroic efforts of immunologists. But the histories are exciting for another reason too. They opened a new development in immunology: restoring immunity to those who are immunologically deficient.

Bone Marrow, Grafts, and Antibodies

Since 1968 immunologists have tried an assortment of treatments for immunodeficient patients. They include bone marrow or fetal liver grafts to restore those stem cells that make the immune system. The fetal liver appears to contain stem cells that later leave it as it matures. Bone marrow or fetal livers are usually given to patients with combined immunodeficiency disease—that is, those who lack both cellular and antibody immunity. Still another treatment that is given is fetal thymus. It is given to patients who lack a thymus or who have defects in cellular immunity. Blood fractions—separated portions—that are rich in antibodies are used as treatment in those patients who lack sufficient antibodies. These treatments have been spectacularly successful in some patients, yet they have failed in many others. Consequently immunologists are trying to overcome certain problems associated with the treatments and to understand better the subtle differences between the diseases. Then they can tailor treatments to these differences.

During the past seven years, for example, 52 attempts to treat immunodeficient patients with bone marrow, fetal liver, or fetal thymus have been reported to the American College of Surgeons/National Institutes of Health Bone Marrow Transplant Registry. Of the 52 patients, only 22 are alive today with functioning grafts. Why did the treatments often fail? One of the major reasons was that the implanted tissues and the recipients' bodies did not have the same transplantation antigens. As in heart and kidney transplants, it was a matter of rejection of tissues that couldn't match chemically. This is the opinion of Dr. Bortin, a consultant to the ACS/NIH marrow transplant registry.

Some of these cases of immunological rejection were "classical" (serving as a model) host-versus-graft rejections, Dr. Bortin explains. In other words, patients had enough immunity to reject the implanted tissues. In certain cases, however, the implanted immunological tissues rejected the patients. This is called graft-versus-host disease. A full-blown graft-versus-host reaction is a frightening thing to observe. It strikes patients in the skin, stomach, liver, and lymph tissues. It can lead swiftly to death unless it is brought under control.

Immunologists are taking various approaches to solving these rejection problems. One approach is to give patients repeated inoculations of small amounts of marrow. The idea here is a sort of sneak-through approach. If marrow is gradually added to a patient's body, then there should be less danger of its rejecting the patient, or of the patient's rejecting it. Another approach is to give recipients immunosuppressive drugs until the dangers of rejection are past. But these drugs subject patients to the danger of uncontrollable infections, just as they do in heart and kidney transplants.

Dr. Joseph Bellanti and his immunology team at Georgetown University Medical School have taken still another route to minimize the danger of rejection in thymus transplants. They put the thymus into a little chamber before it is placed in a patient. The chamber is like a porous membrane. It lets hormones and other chemical substances escape from the thymus and gave a patient cellular immunity. But it also keeps the thymus from having direct contact with the patient's body and trying to destroy it.

Dr. Good is now with the Sloan-Kettering Institute in New York City. He and his team are setting up a data bank of potential bone marrow donors for immunodeficient patients. The potential donors are typed, or classified, for transplantation antigens. The results are fed into a computer. Then if a particular patient needs bone marrow, the computer can find a donor with transplantation antigens that are identical with those of the patient. The chances of finding an ideal donor outside one's immediate family are extremely slim. That is why a large data bank and computer will be so valuable to these patients.

The data bank at Sloan-Kettering is being hooked up with others at the University of Minnesota, Duke University, and with several in Holland, Denmark, and Sweden. The ultimate aim is to have a large international system to find ideal donors.

Still other approaches, more experimental, are being taken to overcome the rejection problems. A few immunologists are trying to separate stem cells from those cells in bone marrow that cause graft-versus-host reactions. They have tried injecting only the stem cells into immunodeficient patients. So far, though, these efforts have not been very successful. Either they have not given patients an immune system, or they have caused a graft-versus-host reaction. One reason the stem cells are not working so well may be that they have not yet been well separated from the other cells.

Dr. Patrica Bealmear and her colleagues at Baylor College of Medicine in Houston have managed to overcome acute graft-versus-host reactions in animals. They first separate out those fragments of antibodies that attack tissue antigens. They inject the fragments into animals that have received bone marrow transplants. The antibody fragments attach themselves to the bone marrow cells and keep the cells from attacking the animals. However, this approach has not yet worked in preventing long-range graft-versus-host disease.

Meanwhile, other immunologists are trying to better understand those diseases for which bone marrow, livers, or thymuses are given. Dr. Rebecca Buckley is a pediatric immunologist with Duke University. She and her colleagues have studied some 40 patients with combined immunodeficiency disease. They have found, contrary to what they expected, that these patients do not lack B and T cells; rather, these cells do not seem to function right. Why not? "A defective enzyme may be the key," Dr. Buckley suggests.

In 1972 Dr. Hilaire Meuwissen of the Albany, New York, Medical Center and his colleagues found that one boy who had combined immunodeficiency disease also lacked an enzyme. This enzyme, called adenosine deaminase, participates in the operations of DNA, the genetic material of cells. Since then, other investigators have found 14 other patients with this disease and who also lack the enzyme.

New Treatments and New Hopes

These discoveries open up new treatment possibilities for combined immunodeficiency disease. For instance, B and T cells can now be grown in the laboratory. Drugs can be tested on them. Perhaps one will be found that can make defective B and T cells function correctly. There is also the possibility that therapy with the adenosine deaminase enzyme might eventually help correct the B and T cell problems. At this time, however, it would be tricky injecting the enzyme into a patient and trying to make sure that the enzyme ends up in the patient's B and T cells, where it is needed.

Still other treatments look promising for defects in cellular immunity. One is transfer factor. As we mentioned, this is being used in the treatment of cancer patients. It is chemical material that is taken from the lymphocytes of persons who have overcome cancer. The material is then injected into a person with cancer in the hope that it will transfer immunity against cancer to the patient. The transfer factor that is used in the treatment of immunodeficient patients is based on a similar principle. It is taken from the lymphocytes of persons with healthy immunity and injected into immunodeficient patients. The substance is helping to improve cellular immunity in some patients, perhaps by helping the patients' T cells reach a state of maturity. However, it is not always successful.

Another treatment that looks promising is one using thymus hormone. A frail five-year-old, Heather, had spent most of her young life ill with one disease or another. She had diarrhea, pneumonia, skin infections. Her thymus was underdeveloped and her T cells could not attack antigens. So Drs. Alan A. Goldstein of the University of Texas at Galveston and Arthur Ammann of the University of California at San Francisco embarked

Dr. Arthur Ammann with Heather, whose thymus gland was improperly developed, giving her a weak immunity against disease. An experimental treatment with a thymus hormone much improved her health.   UNIVERSITY OF CALIFORNIA

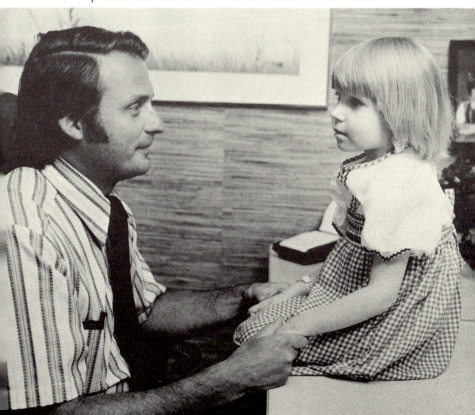

on a novel treatment for Heather. It was thymosin, a hormone from the thymus of the calf. They took some of Heather's T cells and placed them in a test tube in the presence of thymosin. As they hoped, the hormone turned the T cells into immune fighters.

Then the doctors gave Heather thymosin injections. She got an injection each day for 23 days. Her T cells started to fight off the infections in her body. Then she was given injections of thymosin once a week during several more months. Her health continued to improve. Her physicians conclude that thymosin probably helps T cells that are immature to become mature. Transfer factor, on the other hand, passes a specific cellular immunity from the donor to the recipient. But both forms of treatment help restore cellular immunity.

Immunologists are not ignoring antibody deficiencies either. Dr. Fred Rosen and his colleagues at the Children's Hospital Medical Center in Boston have been studying acquired variable hypogammaglobulinemia. "Acquired" means that the disease is not inherited, as most immunodeficiency diseases are. "Variable" means that patients vary in the amount of deficiency they have. "Hypogammaglobulinemia" means that the patients do not make as many antibodies as they need. Consequently the patients have recurrent infections, such as pneumonia. Many also develop arthritis or even cancer. Dr. Rosen and his colleagues have found that all patients with this disease do not necessarily have the same defect. Some have B cells that cannot make antibodies. Others have B cells that can, but these antibodies cannot enter the bloodstream. So Dr. Rosen and his team conclude that this disease consists of defects that occur at various stages as B cells mature into antibody-secreting cells.

Dr. Thomas Waldmann and his colleagues at the National Cancer Institute have also been studying this disease. They have come up with complementary results, finding out that some of the patients with this disease have a superabundance of T cells that suppress B cells. As a result, the patients' B cells cannot make all the antibodies that the patients need.

These new insights into acquired variable hypogammaglobulinemia may lead to more effective treatments for the disease. For instance, Dr. Warren Strober, one of Dr. Waldmann's colleagues, says that it is now possible to study the suppressor T cells in the test tube and to see whether drugs might counter their action. If such a drug is found, it might be given to patients with the disease and allow their B cells to produce enough antibodies. The finding, Dr. Strober says, also shows that bone marrow treatment for this disease is probably not a good idea. If bone marrow is given, the suppressor T cells would suppress the stem cells in the bone marrow.

Still other immunologists are working on improving the diagnosis of immunodeficiency diseases so that treatments can be given earlier to patients and be more effective. Until now, the only way to test infants for antibody deficiencies was to wait until they were old enough to have large samples of blood drawn from them. Now Dr. Stephen H. Polmar, of Case Western Reserve University in Cleveland, has devised a test that requires only a minute sample of blood, and newborns

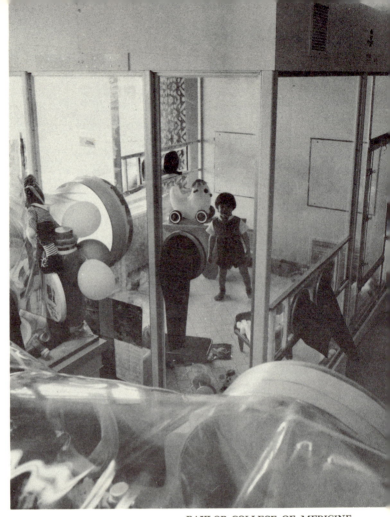

Baby David spent the early part of his life in a germ-free plastic bubble, seen here at the bottom of the picture; now he lives also in the germ-free playroom connected to it by the porthole at left. The black "stockings" allow attendants to manipulate objects inside the room without contaminating it with microbes. David's immunity is almost nonexistent, so he has to live in this protected way until doctors possibly fulfill their hope of giving him normal immunity.

can be screened right away for antibody deficiencies. If they are found to have such deficiencies, they can receive treatment before they become seriously ill.

The lives of some little patients are hanging in the balance until treatments improve. A prime example is Baby David of Houston, Texas. Some years ago a couple in Houston gave birth to Baby David. The doctors had good reason to believe that he had combined immunodeficiency disease. So right after birth he was put in a germ-free plastic bubble. The doctors tested him for the disease. Unfortunately he had it. Baby David was not as lucky as the other two Davids, however. He did not have a brother or sister who had the same transplantation antigens that he did. So they could not give him the bone marrow he needed to correct his immune deficiencies. The doctors tried to find some unrelated person who had identical transplantation antigens, and who could donate bone marrow to him, but without success.

For a long time now, this black-eyed boy with a winning smile has been living in his germ-free bubble. He receives lots of love and attention from his parents and from the hospital staff that takes care of him. In fact, he is a world-wide celebrity. He is the only child who has spent all his life in a bubble. But Baby David is no longer a baby. Perhaps the ideal bone marrow donor will turn up, or some new treatment will solve his immune deficiency problems. Only then will he be able to leave his bubble and safely step into the real, disease-threatening world.

9. THE IMMUNE HORIZON

Mummies buried 2000 years ago in Peru have been found to have the same HL-A antigens that people in Peru have today. This discovery gives archaeologists a better idea of the biology of ancient peoples. It shows how immunological tools can benefit the science of archaeology. . . .

Until recently, immunologists thought that only mammals had immune systems. They have now found that hagfish, sharks, and other animals lower on the evolutionary scale also have immune systems. These systems are more primitive than those of mammals, however. Scientists at San Diego State University are using this discovery to immunize lobsters against diseases. In this way, lobsters that are raised for food can be kept healthy and tasty. . . .

At the University of Chicago, a monkey has kicked his heroin habit. A medical student at the university injected the monkey with antibodies. The antibodies countered the euphoria—an exaggerated elation—and addiction of heroin. This feat opens up the possibility of giving heroin vaccines to heroin addicts, to help them overcome their addiction. . . .

Scientists at Harvard Medical School have managed to do what has never been done before. This is to grow, in the test tube, antibodies that are active against a specific disease. The disease is pneumonia. Antibodies that combat other diseases will probably also be grown in the test tube eventually. When that time comes, doctors will have large amounts of antibodies to use as treatments against specific diseases. . . .

These discoveries and achievements show how explosive the field of immunology is. Month by month—week by week, even—immunological research is being applied to an ever broader spectrum of scientific questions and challenges. As a result it is helping the human race in ways that few people would have dreamed of 10 or 20 years ago. For example, immunologists have started looking at the role of immunity in heart disease, alcoholism, and dental problems.

Heart, Liver, and Teeth

Consider heart attacks. A Harvard University doctor recently observed that complement is a factor in injury to the heart during a heart attack. If complement's participation can be prevented, perhaps heart attacks won't be so severe. British scientists have found that patients who die from heart attacks have an excessive amount of antibodies against milk and egg whites. This finding suggests that foods act as antigens and provoke antibody responses in the body. How antibodies to milk and egg whites might possibly lead to a heart attack, however, remains a mystery.

As far as immunity and alcoholism are concerned, New Mexico physicians have found that there is a marked decrease in the number of T cells in chronic alcoholics with liver disease. But there is no such decrease in chronic alcoholics without liver disease. So the investigators conclude that the reason some alcoholics develop liver disease, and others do not, is a matter of how robust their immune systems are. In short, deficiency in cellular immunity may help trigger alcoholic liver disease.

Macrophages and lymphocytes may contribute to tooth loss among older Americans if tissue culture studies are any indication of what goes on in people's mouths. Macrophages can stimulate the production of an enzyme, collagenase, which leads to the breakdown of the bone and collagen fibers that support teeth. This discovery was made by scientists at the National Institute of Dental Research. Both macrophages and lymphocytes can increase the production of a biological material—called osteoclast-activating factor—that can bring about the loss of bone. This finding comes from the Walter Reed Army Institute of Dental Research.

On the positive side, though, British dentists have found that persons who have few cavities have a lot of antibodies against decay-causing bacteria that affect teeth. Persons with many cavities have few of these antibodies. They seem to inhibit an enzyme that lets the bacteria stick to teeth and cause decay.

Increasing efforts are also being made to diagnose and treat diseases by immunological means. Physicians are now using a technique called immunofluorescence to quickly diagnose viral diseases. Antibodies to a suspect virus are exposed to tissue taken from a patient. If the antibodies attack, the physician can conclude that the patient is infected with the virus in question. This technique gives results in three hours. Other techniques take from one to 20 days.

If a blood clot clogs the lungs, it leads to death. Doctors at the Downstate Medical Center in Brooklyn, New York, have found a means of diagnosing such clots immunologically. They take blood from patients who may have clots and inject it into rabbits. The animals make antibodies to antigens on the clots. Blood from a patient suspected of having a clot is then exposed to the antibodies. If these clump with the blood, it suggests that the patient has a clot.

Immunologists are trying to find out whether the presence of various antibodies in the throat and lungs reflects susceptibility to disease. They have found that raised levels of IgM or IgG antibodies often signify that infection is present. However, raised levels of IgEs usually mean that a patient has allergies.

A Cornell University doctor is exploring the possibility that infections can be detected in unborn babies.

He is measuring the levels of IgA in the amniotic fluid that surrounds the fetus. He is trying to find out what levels of IgA are normal or abnormal at various stages of pregnancy. His findings may then be used to detect the presence of infections in the unborn baby. If a fetus appears to have an infection, doctors can then be ready to treat it as soon as it is born. Eventually doctors may also be able to treat babies before they are born.

Immunological treatments for diseases are also being expanded. Transfer factor is being used to restore immunity against tuberculosis and certain fungus diseases. The World Health Organization is planning a field trial to use transfer factor to treat patients with leprosy. There are more lepers in the world than there are people in New York City—over 10 million. The Rockefeller Foundation is giving transfer factor to Puerto Ricans who have the stubborn tropical disease schistosomiasis. Scientists at Rockefeller University are giving the factor to patients with multiple sclerosis.

In this case lymphocytes are taken from healthy persons who show a lot of immunity to the measles virus. This virus, as we noted, may trigger multiple sclerosis. Transfer factor is extracted from these lymphocytes and injected into multiple-sclerosis victims. It helps the patients' lymphocytes to "recognize" measles virus and has also improved the patients' conditions.

Understanding Vaccines Better

As mentioned earlier, the basic concept of vaccines hasn't really changed much during the past 200 years.

That is, if an infectious organism is injected into a person in minute amounts, it will provoke an antibody response. But it won't give the person a disease. Then, if the person later comes into contact with the organism in the natural environment, he will have already made enough antibodies to fight off the organism. However, recent advances in immunology, chemistry, and genetics are now being pooled to refine this basic vaccine concept.

A promising new mode of vaccine delivery is by nose spray instead of by needle injection. Spray vaccines are being developed for strep throat and German measles. This news should make youngsters of the world stand up and cheer. The Smith, Kline and French Laboratories have received permission to sell, in Belgium, a flu vaccine that can be sprayed up the nose. The vaccine was approved by Belgium authorities. It was made available to Belgians during the 1974-75 flu season. The vaccine will probably be licensed in other countries as well.

Live viruses make ideal vaccines in that they provoke strong antibody responses. But there is always the danger that live viruses might reproduce themselves in people and cause disease. Dead viruses cannot replicate, or reproduce, and cause disease. But they do not stimulate the strong antibody protection that live viruses do. Consequently Dr. Robert Webster, a virologist at St. Jude's Children's Hospital in Memphis, is trying to get the best of both worlds. He is trying to come up with a flu vaccine that will be potent, yet safe. How will he do this? By using only parts of the flu virus as a vaccine.

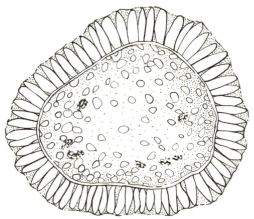

Diagrammatic drawing of a Hong Kong flu virus, based on an electron-microscope photograph. The center contains proteins and pieces of RNA that are thought to control the manufacture of proteins in the virus. The center is surrounded by a double layer of lipids—a group of substances that includes the fats. The rod-shaped spikes pointing outward in this layer attach the virus to a host cell when infection occurs. Scientists have found that flu viruses change the chemical nature of the lipid layer from time to time, which accounts for the fact that epidemics of flu tend to occur rather often, and especially severely in approximate ten-year cycles.

The flu virus is a minute protein sac held together with fats. Inside the sac is the genetic information, in the form of a threadlike molecule of a nucleic acid, that the virus needs to replicate itself. On the surface of the sac are little spikes of protein. These little antigens prompt an immune reaction if the virus is injected into someone. So Dr. Webster is trying to isolate only these antigens to use as a vaccine. In this way he hopes to trigger sharp immunity in people. But there won't be any danger of the flu virus' replicating itself and causing disease.

"A bacterium is a big creature," Dr. Webster explains. "But a virus is tiny. Getting pure antigens from a virus stretches the limits of our technology right now." Unlike viral antigens, bacterial antigens have been used as vaccines since the 1940s. Still, such antigen use is becoming more sophisticated. For instance, some twelve kinds of related bacteria cause most cases of pneumococcal pneumonia. Dr. Robert Austrian of the University of Pennsylvania has designed a pneumonia vaccine that contains antigens from all the crucial bacteria. Clinical trials with this vaccine ran from 1972 to 1975. So far the vaccine appears 80 per cent effective.

A scientist at Rockefeller University has developed a vaccine for meningococcal meningitis. This disease can lead to neurological damage and death among infants. The vaccine consists of two antigens from the bacterium that causes the disease. The vaccine works well in adolescents and adults. But whether it helps infants is not yet certain. There is a good chance that it won't be very helpful. The reason is that infants' immune systems are not mature. So they cannot respond forcefully to vaccine stimulation.

If the vaccine does not protect infants, there may be another way of making it work. And that is by giving infants harmless bacteria along with the vaccine to step up the development of their immune systems. In fact, Dr. John Robbins of the National Institute of Child Health and Human Development is exploring this approach. He took harmless bacteria that live in the human intestine. He fed the bacteria to some human volunteers.

The bacteria stimulated the volunteers' bodies. As a result, the volunteers' tissues produced antibodies that were effective not only against the harmless bacteria but against the meningitis bacteria as well. This happened because meningitis bacteria are similar to those that live in the intestine.

New Viral Vaccines—and Synthetic Ones?

Meanwhile, several other teams are trying to alter the genetics of flu viruses so they might be used as effective and safe flu vaccines. Dr. Ed Kilbourne of the Mount Sinai School of Medicine in New York City mated flu viruses with harmless viruses. He plans to take some of the genetically mixed offspring from the two kinds of viruses and use them as a vaccine. Such a vaccine would confer only partial immunity.

"The point of this," Dr. Kilbourne explains, "is to allow the individual to be infected by the wild flu virus [that which occurs in nature] but not become diseased. The reason is that the best immunity is that which follows natural infection. In other words, we're trying to blunt the effects of natural infection, but not completely prevent it. We want to get the immunizing effects of this infection."

The vaccine looks promising in animal experiments. Dr. Kilbourne is now trying it on human volunteers.

Dr. Fred M. Davenport of the University of Michigan mated different types of flu viruses. He mated them until he got some genetic mutants that thrive at lower tem-

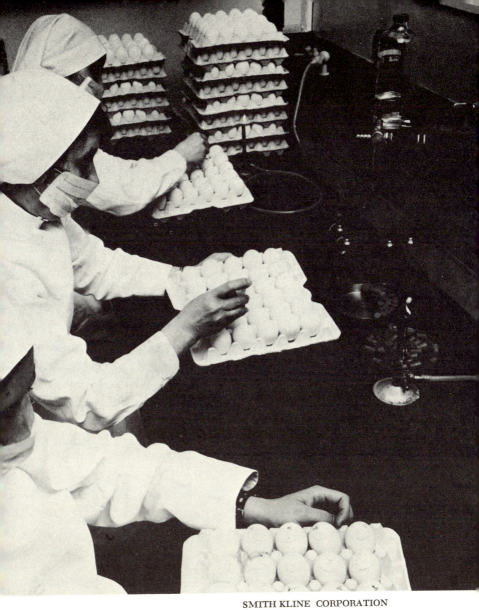

These Belgian technicians are inoculating the developing embryos of chicks with live viruses, a step in producing a live-virus influenza vaccine.

peratures than regular viruses do. He is testing the mutant viruses as a vaccine on volunteers.

Although viruses are not life in the sense that cells are, they can still be "mated," that is, crossed genetically, so that new kinds of viruses with new kinds of genetic material are produced. Viruses are placed in a tissue culture medium and there is some exchange of genetic material. Then the scientist puts antisera in the medium; these inhibit the mutant viruses he does not want and he can select out those mutant viruses that he desires.

The reason Dr. Davenport is using the viruses as a vaccine is this: if a virus is able to resist high temperature when a patient's temperature is high, the virus is able to cause disease. Otherwise, as soon as a patient's temperature went up, it would kill the virus. Therefore, if disease-causing viruses can be found that thrive in relative cold but not in heat, they should stimulate immunity but not cause active disease.

And in a decade or so we may even have access to vaccines that are made purely of synthetic chemicals. Chemical immunologists from Israel joined forces with the Nobel Prize-winning chemist Dr. Christian B. Anfinsen. They made a synthetic copy of a natural protein (a lysozyme from egg white). They injected this copy into rabbits, and the rabbits made antibodies against it. The antibodies were precisely those that rabbits make against the natural protein. Thus it looks as if synthetic copies of bacterial or viral antigens can be made. And they can be used as vaccines against bacteria and viruses. The advantage of using synthetic chemicals as vaccines, Dr. Anfinsen says, is that many vaccines could be given at once.

Other efforts are being made to harness immunity in order to prevent diseases. Interferon, as mentioned before, is made by cells that are attacked by viruses. Interferon tends to protect cells by acting within them. The other immune fighters protect the cells from without. Interferon was discovered in 1957; since then, scientists have hoped that it might be used as a vaccine against the common cold. But for many years they were not able to harvest enough natural interferon to use for immunization trials. Nor did they know its chemical structure. So they could not synthesize it in the test tube and make large batches.

Recently, however, scientists have managed to gather enough interferon to give to volunteers. And it appears that if it is given in large enough amounts, it can prevent colds. Progress is also being made by Dr. Anfinsen in unraveling the chemistry of interferon.

There is also the possibility that in the future infants will be able to be vaccinated even before they are born. This way they'll get a jump on any diseases that may attack them either before or after birth. A team of immunologists at Harvard Medical School immunized female rats with antigen, then mated them. The offspring of these rats produced more antibodies than did the offspring of rats who had not been immunized. The Harvard investigators believe that the reason for this was that they had been immunized before birth. In other words, before the rat pups were born, antigen probably left their mothers' bloodstream, crossed the placenta into the womb and stimulated their developing immune systems.

Now that so much is known about the immune system, scientists are trying to learn how it interacts with other parts of the body. So far, lymphocytes have been found to interact with prostaglandins and catecholamines. Prostaglandins are a sort of local hormones; that is, they transmit "messages" to cells that are near them. Catecholamines are chemicals that conduct nerve impulses between nerves. Cyclic AMP, a chemical that transmit "messages" within cells, appears capable of inhibiting lymphocytes.

Still one other important trend is emerging on the immune horizon. Immunological tools are being used to better understand various parts of the body. Much has been learned about the role of hormones by removing the glands responsible for their secretion. But many glands secrets more than one hormone. Thus it is desirable to selectively prevent the secretion of a single hormone, or two or three, in order to study others made by the same gland. Antibodies can now be made against hormones. So this approach can be taken.

Antibodies can also be made to block genes or specific parts of genes. This makes it possible to learn more about the actions of neighboring genes.

What will immunological research serve up by the year 2000? A 76-year-old surgeon who has been practicing medicine half a century is willing to make some predictions. He is Dr. Alton Ochsner of New Orleans.

Dr. Ochsner predicts that doctors will be able to manipulate the body's immune system in order to switch off cancer or to let an implanted organ take. Transplantation of organs that now make difficulty, such as livers and lungs, will be routine. But people won't need heart transplants. If their hearts wear out, they will get artificial hearts. "The enormously complex immune processes are yielding rapidly to investigation," Dr. Ochsner says. "It is only a matter of time, and not much time, before we learn to control them."

10. IMMUNITY AND ALL OF US

It was a brisk autumn afternoon in Kentucky. The air was pungent with burning leaves. The ripe persimmons were sweet to the taste. Usually autumn is my favorite time of year. But this particular Saturday I had a headache and felt tired. The doorbell rang. A woman was making a survey to see what aspirin people prefer. She asked me whether I had a preference. I replied that I rarely took aspirin. Then I remembered: that morning I had taken several—which was out of character for me.

That day, and that particular incident, are as fresh in my memory as they were 18 years ago. It was the start of an illness that could have left me paralyzed for life, or even dead.

Events that followed the aspirin woman's departure are rather vague in my mind. My head ached. My body ached. My stomach was upset. I went to bed. My homework for my high school class would have to wait. A fever racked my body, soaring to 103, 104 degrees. My parents called our family doctor. He stopped by to see me on his way home. I became delirious. He ordered me taken to the hospital.

Memories of my hospital stay are dimmer still, except for singular incidents that still stand out with alarming clarity. A nurse jammed a needle into the tip of my finger and withdrew a full test tube of blood. A doctor jammed a needle into my spine and withdrew fluid. I realized that the blood and spinal fluid were needed for tests to find out what was wrong with me. But the pain from those needles was excruciating. In fact, I have never experienced such pain since.

The furrowed brow of our doctor . . . The distressed faces of my mother and father . . . A needle carrying nutrients into a vein in my arm . . . And the realization that I was seriously ill; in fact, that I might die. Curiously, I accepted this possibility without fear. I did regret, however, that I might live to be only 15.

How many days was I in the hospital? I'm not sure. Perhaps a week or two. But toward the latter part of my stay, my fever subsided. The demons flogging my body with pain stole away. My delirum lifted like a fog. I was 10 pounds lighter and incredibly weak. But so thankful! I was going to live after all. Undoubtedly several factors were responsible for my victory over the enemy—excellent medical care, the love of my parents, and of course a robust immune system.

Only after I was back home and on the road to recovery did our doctor tell us what had happened. I had barely escaped the full effects of an illness that could have killed me, or at best left me practically unable to move. The illness, our doctor said, seemed by the symptoms and tests to be infectious polyneuritis. If a patient survives the acute phase, permanent paralysis or even death can strike. The cause of the disease is probably a virus; doctors are not sure. A large concentration of protein in the spinal fluid is one sign that the disease is present. In my case—though this could not be absolutely proved—it is rather likely that I did have the disease and that my body fought it off.

So now, 18 years later, I look back thoughtfully on this one serious illness of my life. If I hadn't inherited a basically healthy body, and if my immune system hadn't been strong, I would be in a miserable state today, if I were alive at all. My bout with illness impressed on me something I had ignored before: the preciousness of good health, and how important it is to take care of one's body, even if its immune system is at its peak.

There are things that all of us can do to keep our immune systems in their best possible condition. One is to eat intelligently. There is ample evidence that diet influences the immune system. Antibodies, lymphocytes, and macrophages are hungry for protein. Deficiencies of this substance decrease both antibody and cellular immunity. Such deficiencies also impair the thymus.

Vitamin A has been found to enhance immunity. Vitamin C seems to be capable of preventing colds, though argument over this may continue a long time. This vitamin tends to make harmless any pollen, dust, foods, and other substances that cause allergies. Iron also seems to be crucial for the immune system. Persons lacking iron have weakened lymphocytes and macrophages. When they eat more iron, their immunity improves.

What Should We Eat?

So what should one eat to protect the immune system? Plently of protein and a variety of vitamins and minerals. A deficiency in even one nutrient probably hurts one's immune forces. Foods that are rich in protein include meat, poultry, fish, and dairy products. Foods that are rich in vitamins and minerals are fruits, vegetables, and whole-grain cereals and breads. Yogurt keeps the harmless bacteria in the stomach and intestines healthy, and these bacteria can keep the immune system primed against harmful bacteria.

Dr. Buckley, mentioned before, is also the mother of four teenagers. She and her husband (also a physician) give their youngsters guidance in their eating habits. "We try to keep them away from sweets and breakfast cereals that are like sweetened candy," she says. "Whole grain cereals are best." Several years ago, whole grain breads and cereals usually had to be bought in health food stores. Now they are sold in supermarkets as well. The reason is that more people realize how healthful and tasty they are and want to buy them.

Another way to keep the immune system strong is to keep skin clean. Skin is one of the body's greatest barriers against attacking bacteria and viruses. This advice comes from Dr. Bellanti, mentioned earlier, who

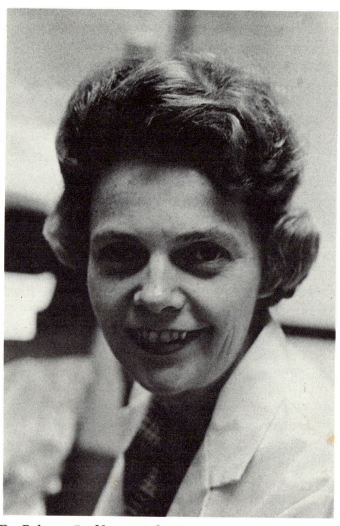

Dr. Rebecca Buckley of Duke University is doing outstanding work in helping youngsters with immunodeficiency diseases. As both a physician and a mother she also has realistic ideas about good food and "junk food."

is the father of seven youngsters and much concerned about what young people can do to stay healthy.

What About Vaccination?

Vaccination against infectious diseases is important. The following are the kinds of vaccinations one should get at various ages, according to the American Academy of Pediatrics:

2 months:
> a diphtheria-tetanus-whooping cough vaccine;
> an oral polio virus vaccine;

4 months:
> a diphtheria-tetanus-whooping cough vaccine;
> an oral polio virus vaccine;

6 months:
> a diphtheria-tetanus-whooping cough vaccine;
> an oral polio virus vaccine;

1 year:
> measles, German measles, and mumps vaccine;

18 months:
> diphtheria-tetanus-whooping cough vaccine;
> an oral polio virus vaccine;

4 to 6 years:
> diphtheria-tetanus-whooping cough vaccine;
> an oral polio virus vaccine;

14 to 16 years:
> tetanus-diphtheria vaccine, adult type;

every 10 years thereafter:
> the same.

A female of child-bearing age who has never been vaccinated against German measles should have a blood test to see whether she is immune to this disease. If not, she should have the vaccine for it. With this treatment, any child she may bear will not be vulnerable to the German measles virus, which can seriously damage unborn babies.

People traveling outside the continental United States must have certain vaccinations, depending on where they plan to go. Public health departments have the complete, up-to-date information on what inoculations are a must. Pregnant women who plan to travel to certain areas of the world require very special immunizing planning by a doctor. Not all kinds of vaccination are entirely safe during pregnancy. That is why the woman who is considering traveling abroad or to any place where vaccinations may be required should see her physician as soon as possible if she is in any stage of pregnancy.

Finally, where there is a threat of epidemic or outbreak of any communicable disease, the wise course is to consult one's doctor or local health department to learn whether to have a vaccination or an injection of gamma globulin for protection.

Moderate exercise helps too; it brings blood to the lymph tissues. Scottish immunologists have found that exercise rapidly activates B cells. However, exercise does not seem to have much effect on T cells. Regular sleeping habits and adequate sleep can also benefit one's immune system. The immune fighters, as was pointed out in Chapter 2, are probably most susceptible to infections from three to four in the morning. And during one's active hours the body should not be exposed to too much physical stress; excesses of cold, heat, and exercise can impair the immune system. According to Dr. Hans Selye, a well known stress scientist, one should also try to avoid negative mental stressors such as tension, emotional upsets, insecurity, and aimlessness—difficult though that usually is to accomplish. Such strains too can weaken immunity. They have been found to lead to headaches, ulcers, heart attacks, and even mental illness. Emotional upsets often precede illnesses in young people. Some stress in life is not only necessary, but desirable, Dr. Selye says. The danger comes from *too much*.

Before anyone takes up smoking—whether regular cigarettes or marijuana—he or she should consider the fact that smoking depresses the immune fighters, including the macrophages. Cigarette smokers lose more work days than nonsmokers because of flu, bronchitis, and other diseases. Regular marijuana smoking has been found in several studies to impair the B and T cells.

Is there any simple formula for keeping your immune system in tip-top shape? Yes, there is. It is to *live fully, but in moderation*. This is the advice of Dr. Irving Page, editor of the magazine *Modern Medicine*. It is also the advice of Dr. Jonas Salk, discoverer of the Salk polio vaccine. Dr. Selye suggests that one's aim in life should be to express oneself as fully as possible, but to be sure to find one's own level of maximum stress.

GLOSSARY

allergy: An adverse immunological reaction to any number of substances.

anaphylaxis: An overwhelming allergic reaction.

asthma: A disease of the lungs that cuts off breathing.

antibody: A kind of protein that is made by cells (B cells) that come from bone marrow. It protects the human body against infectious agents. It also plays a role in cancer, allergies, and organ transplants.

antigen: Anything that the imune system considers foreign. It can be a virus, bacterium, or molecules of such an organism.

autoimmunity: Immunity against oneself.

bacterium: A minute, primitive cell. A number of bacteria cause diseases.

B cell: A cell that comes from bone marrow and that makes antibodies.

BCG: The tuberculosis vaccine. BCG is being used as one kind of immunotherapy for cancer.

blocking antibody: An antibody, or part of an antibody, that protects a tumor rather than rejects it; or that protects an implanted organ rather than rejects it.

bone marrow: Connective tissue in the core of bones. It gives rise to the body's immune system.

catecholamine: A chemical that conducts nerve impulses between nerves.

cell: The smallest basic unit of life. A bacterium is a cell. A human is made up of some 100 trillion cells.

cellular immunity: Immunity provided by a kind of cell known as the T cell (from the thymus gland).

cyclic AMP: A chemical that transmits information within cells.

chromosome: A threadlike part of the nucleus of a cell; it contains DNA.

complement: A kind of protein that assists in the immune system's battle against antigens. The complement group consists of nine, possibly 11, different proteins.

DNA: A molecule that contains the genetic information of a cell. Molecules of DNA make up genes, which are distributed through each chromosome.

enhancing antibody: See blocking antibody.

enzyme: A protein that speeds up a chemical reaction in a cell without becoming a part of the reaction.

gamma globulin: The part of blood that is rich in antibodies.

HL-A antigens: Antigens on the surface of cells that lead to rejection of a transplanted organ.

humoral immunity: Immunity provided by antibodies.

hormone: A chemical messenger, or mediator, of the body. It is made by certain cells, then acts on other cells that are far away.

immune memory: Once the immune fighters of the body overcome an infectious organism, they will be particularly prepared to kill it the next time they meet it; this is immune memory.

immune system: The system of the body that protects the body from anything it considers foreign and a threat.

immunity: Protection.

immunization: Injecting a little bit, or a weakened form, of an infectious organism into a person to stimulate immunity against the organism, without causing disease. Vaccination.

immunodeficiency: A condition in which some aspect of the immune response is weak or absent.

immunogeneticist: A scientist who studies the genes that make the immune fighters and that control their actions.

immunoglobulin: A class of protein. All antibodies are immunoglobulins. But all immunoglobulins are not necessarily antibodies.

immunologist: A scientist who studies the immune system.

interferon: A group of proteins made by cells that are attacked by a cold virus or other infectious agent. It tends to protect the cells from the agent working within the attacked cells rather than outside them.

lymphocyte: A kind of white cell that gives immune protection to the body.

lymph tissue: Tissue that contains a colorless fluid called lymph. It is rich in B and T cells.

lysosomal enzymes: Enzymes made by little sacs in a macrophage called lysosomes.

macrophage: A type of white cell, one of the immune fighters.

parasite: An organism that takes nourishment from its host. The parasite is one of the infectious agents that the immune fighters attack.

platelets: Fragments from the bone marrow that aid in clotting blood.

polypeptide chain: The basic component of an antibody (or of any protein).

prostaglandin: A chemical that transmits information to nearby cells.

protein: A molecule made of polypeptide chains, and made by the cell. Proteins do many things for cells and tissues.

RNA: A molecule that translates the genetic information in a DNA molecule into protein manufacture.

spleen: An organ near the stomach. It is rich in T and B cells.

stem cells: Specialized cells in bone marrow. Stem cells make red blood cells, white blood cells, and platelets.

slow virus: A virus that damages the body over a period of months or years.

T cell: A lymphocyte that is processed by the thymus. T cells provide cellular immunity.

thymin: A hormone from the thymus of the calf.

thymus: A small gland near the heart. It turns lymphocytes into T cells.

tissue: A group of cells that carries out some special function in the body.

tonsil: A mass of lymphoid tissue on each side of the throat. It is rich in B and T cells.

transfer factor: Chemical material taken from lymphocytes that have shown strong resistance to a particular disease. The material can then be injected into a person and transfer cellular immunity appropriate for that disease.

vaccine: A bit of a disease-causing organism that is injected into a person to give him immunity against a disease. *See* immunization.

virus: A minute core of genetic material surrounded by proteins and fats.

SUGGESTED READING

Younger Books

Irmengarde Eberle, *Modern Medical Discoveries* (T. Y. Crowell, N.Y., 1968). Has a chapter on vaccines against infectious diseases and cancer.

James Hemming, *Mankind Against the Killers* (Longmans, Green, N.Y., 1956). About infectious diseases and efforts to find drugs to fight them. Includes a chapter on vaccines.

David C. Knight, *Your Body's Defenses* (McGraw-Hill, N.Y., 1975). Mechanisms acting against accidents and infectious diseases.

Fred Reinfeld, *Miracle Drugs and the New Age of Medicine* (Sterling, N.Y., 1962). About infectious diseases, drugs, and vaccines.

Sarah Riedman, *Shots Without Guns* (Rand McNally, Skokie, Ill., 1960). The history of vaccination, from Edward Jenner to Jonas Salk and Albert Sabin, creators of the polio vaccines.

Tony Simon, *The Heart Explorers* (Basic Books, N.Y., 1966). A history of heart surgery. Includes several chapters on heart transplants and their imunological problems. There is also mention of Charles Hufnagel, one of the pioneers in heart transplants.

Older and Adult Books

Harold Smeck, *Immunology: The Many-Edged Sword* (George Braziller, N.Y., 1974). Essays on different areas of immunological research—use of immunization to prevent blood incompatibility between mother and child; how doctors are manipulating the immune system to cope with disease; the immunological problems of organ transplantation; etc.

David Wilson, *Body and Antibody: A Report on the New Immunology* (Alfred A. Knopf, 1972). All about historical and modern immunological research—from early efforts at vaccination to immunological treatments for cancer and other diseases.

INDEX

smoke, 86
Sokal, Dr. Joseph, 77
spleen, 13, 33, 41
staph infection vaccine, 56
stem cells, 15, 20, 21, 41, 115, 116, 118, 120
strep throat, 56, 133
stress, 149
Strober, Dr. Warren, 125
Strom, Dr. Terry, 105, 106
sumac, 86
syphilis vaccine, 56

T cells, 15, 16, 18, 19, 20, 21, 22, 23, 24, 26, 30, 32, 36, 38, 39, 40, 41, 43, 46, 58, 59, 60, 63, 65 69, 74, 76, 88, 91, 92, 93, 97, 108, 109, 111, 121, 122, 123, 124, 125, 130, 148
Temin, Dr. Howard M., 72
Terasaki, Dr. Paul I., 105
tetanus vaccine, 56, 147
thymin, 21
thymosin, 124
thymus, 15, 20, 21, 30, 39, 40, 41, 93, 118, 120, 123, 141
thymus hormone treatment, 123; *see also* thymin *and* thymosin
thymus transplants, 118, 120
titration analysis, 98
tonsils, 18, 43, 45
toxemia of pregnancy, 38
toxoplasma, 59
toxoplasmosis, 59, 60
transfer factor, 79, 80, 122, 124, 132
transplantation antigens, 119, 120, 127

tropical diseases, 66, 67, 69
trypanosome, 59
tuberculin skin test, 57
tuberculosis, 12, 56, 69, 77, 80, 132
tuberculosis antigen, 80
tuberculosis bacteria, 57, 78
tumbleweed, 86
tumor cells, 74, 76, 79
tumor-cell injections, 79
tumors, 73, 74, 78, 79, 81, 83
typhus vaccine, 56

ulcers, 145

vaccination, 54; *see also* immunization
vaccines, 56, 57, 69, 77, 132, 136, 138, 147, 148; *see also specific vaccines*
Vibrio comma, 55
viruses, 14, 49, 57, 59, 83, 90, 94, 131, 133, 134, 135, 138, 139, 144, 145; *see also specific viruses and categories*
vitamins, 48, 144

Waldmann, Dr. Thomas, 125
warts, 57, 64
wasps, 85, 86, 96
Webster, Dr. Robert, 133, 135
whooping cough vaccine, 56, 147
Wilson, Dr. Raphael, 6

X-rays, 72

Zigas, Dr. Victor, 60, 62